OBESITY

CAUSES & CONSEQUENCES

PATRICK WULF HANSON

PATRICK WULF HANSON

OBESITY

CAUSES & CONSEQUENCES

Acknowledgements

I would like to express my deepest gratitude to my friend and colleague, Dr. Frederik Persson, who was instrumental in providing a thorough and crucial scientific evaluation of the contents of this book. Your encouraging feedback is not only valuable for this book, but has also proved to be extremely valuable for the planned second volume, covering prevention and treatment of obesity.

I would also like to thank Emil Thorsson at Grafikhuset.se for helping me present the book in its cool layout, and Lise Gottlieb for valuable help and support in getting it published.

Finally, I would like to express my deepest gratitude to my wife, Katja Wulf Hanson. Your never failing support and spot-on feedback has been absolutely crucial in my work with this book.

Without all the valuable support and input I have received from all of you this book would never have been completed.

Foreword

Let there be no doubt, obesity is a threat to mankind. It has the potential to be the plague of our time, and for the first time in history life expectancy may decrease due to this feature of western developed lifestyle. Only in recent years has the true global scale of this condition has been realised.

Through decades of research an understanding of the pathophysiology has been developed, but many unsolved issues remain, and more work is needed to uncover the many causes of obesity.

In such a vast area with many contributions it can seem impossible to get an overview of the pathophysiology, epidemiology and obesity-associated conditions and complications.

In this book, Patrick Wulf Hanson accomplishes just that. Overall, this is a thorough, methodological and comprehensive overview of available knowledge on the matter. In addition, it is written in a form and language that will suit scientists, medical professionals or science students at several levels.

I recommend this book for anyone looking for an extensive introduction to and an overview of a health care issue that affects us all.

Prof. Peter Rossing
Chief Physician, DMSc, Steno Diabetes Center

INTRODUCTION AND DEFINITIONS
OF OVERWEIGHT & OBESITY

The complexity of obesity is confirmed by the fact that we have not yet managed to figure out how to best prevent or cure it. It has been a big problem for a long time, and it continues to be bigger problem that, if we don't figure it out, will become incomprehensible.

This book is suitable for healthcare professionals, such as doctors, nurses, scientists, students, etc., looking for a summarised, yet comprehensible, overview of obesity, its causes and consequences.

A major breakthrough in medicine occurred in 2013 when the American Medical Association (AMA) officially recognised obesity as a disease[1]. The desired outcome is that this initiative will minimise the obesity consequences by encouraging healthcare providers to put more emphasis on the effects of obesity.

Hopefully many countries will follow AMA's example to proactively treat obesity, as the problem is extremely serious and the future health and financial consequences are incomprehensible.

One of our basic survival skills is easting. Eating is normally considered a good thing, but unfortunately over the last 30 years this has changed and our eating habits are slowly killing us. Excessive eating is thus not equivalent with improved survival.

The increase and easy availability of cheap and unhealthy fast-food choices is no doubt contributing to the problem. Excessive eating which leads to storing of energy, combined with a minimum of physical activity, that is not using enough of the stored energy, will unsurprisingly lead to an accumulation of both fat and sugar in the body.

Obesity is associated with a significant increase in many other diseases and conditions, as well as higher mortality[2]. Associated disorders include diabetes mellitus, hypertension, dyslipidaemia, heart disease, stroke, sleep apnoea, cancer, and many other serious conditions. In 2013 the World Health Organization (WHO) reported that more than 1.5 billion adults aged 20 and over were overweight in 2008, and 200 million men and nearly 300 million women were found to be obese[3].

More than 40 million children under the age of five were overweight in 2011. The same report presents that 65% of the world's population live in countries where overweight and obesity kills more people than underweight[3].

This is extra scary when you consider obesity is preventable! As an example, sticking to a healthy diet and lifestyle can prevent as many as four out of five heart attacks in men[4]. On top of this, it is estimated that the overall economic burden of obesity in the Unites States alone amounts to $215 billion[5].

Social and emotional consequences of obesity affect most age and socioeconomic groups around the world, but the consequences and implications are more serious in the developing countries[6]. In 1997 obesity was formally classified as a pandemic by the WHO[7].

Genes also play an important role in determining obesity[8]. This is clearly confirmed in people who eat healthy food and exercise regularly but still gain weight easier, and have a harder time losing it compared to others who follow the same diet and exercise plan.

Similarly, environmental factors have great influence on obesity. This is confirmed by the drastic changes seen during the last 30 years where more time is spent on sitting in front of a TV or computer, driving instead of walking or cycling, eating bigger portions of food containing too much sugar and fat, and at the same time devoting less time for physical activity[9]

The substantially increased risk of developing a number of serious conditions, and the large increase of these conditions has become a serious and significantly rising public health problem[10-13].

Publications by large organisations, such as the WHO and the National Heart, Lung, and Blood Institute agree on the classifications and definitions of overweight and obesity[14].

Body mass index (BMI)

The rate of obesity is easily determined by calculating body mass index (BMI), which is calculated as weight in kilograms divided by height in metres squared.

Although it is not entirely accurate, the BMI is the most frequently used measure to identify and quantify obesity. BMI is the accepted standard measure for adults and children two years and older, and is considered the most practical way to evaluate overweight and obesity[15].

Therefore, obesity is often assessed by means of indirect estimates of body fat, rather than including other issues relevant to child and adolescent obesity, that is family, schools, health professionals, government, industry and media[16].

Simply put, overweight means an excess of body weight, which is not necessarily caused by fat. However, the word obesity means an excess of fat[14]. Lean and muscular people can thus be overweight, but they can only be obese if they also have too much body fat.

BMI is therefore not a perfect measure since the weight of the calculation does not distinguish between excessive body fat and lean muscle mass. But the likelihood of classifying an athlete with high levels of lean muscle and low levels of body fat as having high BMI by mistake is probably very low.

A more reliable method that measures the regional fat distribution is the waist-to-hip ratio, which is also considered a better measure to predict cardiometabolic risk factors[17]. However, the BMI classification is still regarded as a valuable tool to determine the risk of developing a number of serious conditions that come from obesity[2].

The WHO defines adults with a BMI of 25 or higher as being overweight whereas a BMI of 30 or higher is considered being obese[18]. Contrary to BMI in adults, it varies according to age and sex in children since boys and girls grow and mature differently[19]. As a result, a different reference value has been defined for children[20].

BMI values vary between countries and cultures and in 2009 the United States took the undesirable first position in the global obesity prevalence among the 194 WHO member nations[21].

The International Classification of adult underweight, overweight and obesity according to BMI[22]:

CLASSIFICATION	BMI (KG/M2) PRINCIPAL CUT-OFF POINTS	BMI (KG/M2) ADDITIONAL CUT-OFF POINTS
UNDERWEIGHT	<18.50	<18.50
Severe thinness	<16.00	<16.00
Moderate thinness	16.00 - 16.99	16.00 - 16.99
Mild thinness	17.00 - 18.49	17.00 - 18.49
NORMAL RANGE	18.50 - 24.99	18.50 - 22.99 | 23.00 - 24.99
OVERWEIGHT	≥25.00	≥25.00
Pre-obese	25.00 - 29.99	25.00 - 27.49 | 27.50 - 29.99
OBESE	≥30.00	≥30.00
Obese class I	30.00 - 34.99	30.00 - 32.49 | 32.50 - 34.99
Obese class II	35.00 - 39.99	35.00 - 37.49 | 37.50 - 39.99
Obese class III	≥40.00	≥40.00

BACKGROUND OF
OVERWEIGHT AND OBESITY

Family

Overweight and obesity can occur at any age, but there are certain times in life when weight gain often occurs. This also varies between men and women.

Women naturally gain weight during pregnancy and this may significantly influence body size, shape, and also the subsequent body composition of the child. High BMI before pregnancy and considerable weight gain during pregnancy are considered high risk factors for childhood obesity[23].

Smoking during pregnancy and having diabetes also increases the risk of the child becoming overweight and obese[24-26]. Birth weight itself is not a good predictor of future obesity, but small children, short stature, or a less than average head circumference are better indicators of developing abdominal fatness and other obesity-related conditions later in life[27].

The correlation between the birth weights of twins is similar, but thereafter the weights of identical twins become similar whereas those of dizygotic twins doesn't[28]. Children born by mothers with diabetes are also at higher risk of becoming overweight both as children and adults[29].

Breastfeeding is suggested to be associated with a lower risk of overweight and obesity compared to babies receiving formula[30,31]. Also, children who are breastfed for 12 months or more results in very low obesity rates at school entry[32], confirming that a longer duration of breastfeeding decreases the risk of overweight later in life[33].

If one or both parents are obese children under the age of 3 years are at greater risk of becoming obese as adults compared with children of non-obese parents[34]. The older an obese child becomes, the greater the risk of staying or becoming obese as an adult becomes. Obesity in adolescence is thus closely associated with severe obesity in adults[35].

Not surprisingly, the weight of adolescents is an important indicator for a number of serious health issues during adulthood[36]. In spite of the importance of childhood and adolescent weight, it is clear that most overweight people develop their problem in adult life[37].

Since obesity is classified as a disease, severe obesity in children and adolescents needs to be re-addressed to secure a crystal clear understanding. The current definition is used because it is clinically practical, but only about 4% of children in the US are severely obese[38,39].

This group, however, are at significantly higher risk of developing cardiovascular problems and for developing obesity, or staying obese, in adulthood[38]. The degree of risk associated with overweight is related to the BMI.

The above defines medically significant obesity in children and adolescents. Adolescents with this severe degree of obesity should be treated by a multidisciplinary paediatric weight management team, which may include consideration for weight loss surgery to avoid as many future complications as possible[40].

Lifestyle

Leading an inactive lifestyle inevitably decreases the energy consumption and subsequently promotes overweight and obesity. Several observations illustrate the importance of decreased energy expenditure in the pathogenesis of weight gain. Estimates of calorie intake versus energy consumption suggest that reduced energy expenditure is more important than increased food intake in causing obesity[41].

Another study found that the decline in energy expenditure accounted for almost all of the weight gain [42]. Low levels of physical activity are strongly related to weight gain in both men and women, according to a study that investigated if low, medium and high levels of recreational activity was inversely related to body weight.

The study concluded that both men and women in the low activity category were about 3-4 times more likely to suffer from significant weight gain than the more active subjects[43]. Excessive TV watching appears to be the most predictive behaviour of obesity and diabetes risk. One study concluded that TV was associated with a 23% increase in the risk of obesity and a 14% increase in the risk of diabetes[44]. Less risk was seen with other types of inactive behaviour, such as sitting at work.

Television viewing is perhaps the best established environmental influence on the development of obesity during childhood. The amount of time spent on watching television is directly related to the prevalence of diabetes[44] and obesity in children and adolescents[45-49].

The effects may persist into adulthood. In two studies, television viewing at ≥5 years was independently associated with increased BMI at age 26 to 30 years[50,51]. Other studies suggest that the association between television viewing and obesity is considerably weaker[52-54].

There are several proposed mechanisms for this association in terms of displacement of physical activity, depression of metabolic rate and adverse effects on diet quality[55-58].

One study provides evidence that the effects of television on obesity are mediated primarily by changes in energy intake[57]. Similar associations between television viewing and energy intake have been shown in studies of non-overweight adolescents[59]. The use of electronic games has also been associated with obesity during childhood[60].

In the few studies that analyse the influences separately, the association with obesity is not as strong for electronic games compared with TV[60-62], possibly since the games lack food advertising. A few video games have been specifically designed to provide nutritional education and encourage healthy habits[63,64]. Activity-enhancing games lead to a small to moderate increase in energy consumption while playing[65-69].

Two studies of activity games revealed that energy consumption while playing the games was not as high as playing the actual sport[67,70], and the energy consumption depends on the game played[71].

However, no long-term effect on obesity status could be reported in one study since the use of the games often declined over time[72], while another study reported clinically significant reductions in BMI among young people in a 10-week obesity management program[73].

Obesity is also more prevalent in adults with physical disabilities. Those with impaired lower extremity mobility are at highest risk[74].

Sleep and sleep deprivation

Several studies suggest a link between sleep deprivation and obesity or insulin resistance[75-80], where the effects are reported to be more obvious in heavier children[81]. This has also been confirmed in adults[82]. However, many studies have also suggested that the association may be causal[83-87].

Another large longitudinal study using self-report measures of sleep patterns could not confirm the association between short sleep duration and development of childhood obesity[88]. Intermittent hypoxaemia caused by sleep disordered breathing has been shown to be associated with decreased insulin sensitivity in adolescents, independent of obesity[89,90].

The possible association of alterations in serum leptin and ghrelin levels, both of which have been implicated in the regulation of appetite, or perhaps a longer opportunity to ingest food, need to be further explored.

Smoking and smoking cessation

Smoking cessation is often associated with weight gain, possibly due to the withdrawal of nicotine. The average weight gain has been reported to be 4 to 5 kg, but can be much greater[91,92]. The effects of weight gain and smoking cessation have been studied in identical twins and have shown that smokers were lighter than were nonsmokers suggesting that genetic and environmental factors can be eliminated as the cause of weight gain[93].

Therefore, a diet with decreased calories is recommended to both people who plan to stop smoking and to people who have stopped smoking[94].

Diet, eating, drinking, and the environment

Almost all obesity in children is strongly influenced by environmental factors, caused by either a sedentary lifestyle or a caloric intake that is greater than needs.

The contributions of specific environmental influences are the subject of considerable discussion and research. Environmental factors explain only part of obesity risk, but are important targets for treatment because they are potentially modifiable[95,96].

Increasing trends in glycaemic index of foods, such as sugar-containing beverages, portion sizes, fast-food service, and decreasing physical activity, increasing use of computer-oriented activity, including availability of sidewalks and playgrounds etc., have all been considered as causal influences on the rise in obesity[75,96].

In particular, a number of well-designed studies have shown associations between intake of sugar-containing beverages or low physical activity and obesity or metabolic abnormalities[97-104].

Fructose has increasingly been used as a sweetener since the introduction of high-fructose corn syrups in the 1960s[105,106]. High intake of fructose is also associated with both altered appetite and obesity[107].

Results of individual studies testing interventions to prevent childhood obesity are variable. It is difficult to draw firm conclusions from the literature because interventions tested vary in form and intensity, the populations studied are heterogeneous and subject to selection bias, and there are many potential unmeasured confounders that could affect weight outcomes.

Moreover, it appears that effects of lifestyle interventions on body mass index (BMI) are small at best, with substantial variation, and thus are not detectable without very large sample sizes. Despite these limitations, meta-analyses conclude that interventions to prevent childhood obesity are generally effective[108].

One meta-analysis reported that children enrolled in intervention groups had a mean reduction in adiposity as compared to control groups[108]. While the reported effect was small, this represents a clinically important difference across a population.

The best supported strategies were school-based programs that enhance physical activity, nutrition education, and high quality of food served at school, as well as parent-focused interventions designed to encourage children to be more active and reduce screen time.

Studies targeting younger children (ages 6 to 12 years) were most effective. Because the intervention strategies and results varied widely among the included studies, the effect of each intervention component is not clear.

Many people have a pattern of conscious limitation of food intake, termed restrained eating[109]. This restraint pattern is common in many, if not most, middle-aged women who are of "normal weight".

It may also account for the inverse relationship between bodyweight and social class. Women of higher socioeconomic status more often maintain their weight.

Overeating relative to energy expenditure will uniformly cause obesity[110]. Most obese subjects have lost control of their eating (disinhibition)[111]. The relationship between the frequency of meals and the development of obesity is unsettled.

A five meal-a-day pattern was associated with significantly lower risk of overweight and obesity in a Finnish birth cohort[112] and in a German cohort of younger children[113]. Eating breakfast is associated with lower risk of overweight[114].

One explanation of the effects of frequent small meals versus a few large meals could be the difference in insulin secretion associated with these meal sizes[115].

Epidemiological data suggest that a diet high in fat is associated with obesity. The relative weight in several populations, as an example, is directly related to the percentage of fat in their diets[116].

In a large prospective evaluation of three cohorts, increased consumption of potato chips, potatoes, sugar-sweetened beverages, unprocessed red meat, and processed meats was directly associated with weight gain[117]. In contrast, intake of vegetables, whole grains, fruits, nuts, and yoghurt are inversely associated with weight gain.

There may also be an interaction between dietary habits and a genetic predisposition for obesity[118,119].

As an example, in an evaluation of 32 body mass index (BMI) loci associated with obesity in two large prospective cohort studies, there was an interaction between the genetic predisposition score and the intake of sugar-sweetened beverages, such that adults with a higher genetic predisposition score appeared to be more susceptible on BMI to the adverse effects of sugar-sweetened beverages[118].

Accumulating evidence suggests that consumption of sugar-sweetened beverages (including fruit juice) is an important contributor to the development of obesity in some individuals. According to nationally representative surveys of children in the United States, sugar-sweetened beverages supplied an average of 270 calories per day, representing 10 to 15% of total caloric intake[120].

Moreover, a randomised trial demonstrated that reducing

consumption of sugar-sweetened beverages among overweight and obese adolescents is associated with a modest decrease in BMI[121].

In a separate randomised trial in children aged 5 to 12 years (primarily normal-weight), consumption of one serving of artificially sweetened beverage daily was associated with less weight gain and fat accumulation as compared with consumption of a sugar-sweetened beverage[122].

Finally, in a large observational study in adults, the association between obesity and sugar-sweetened beverages appeared to be mediated in part by genetic factors, which were quantified by a "genetic-predisposition" score, based on 32 BMI-associated loci[118]. In each of these studies, the observed effect sizes were small.

Nonetheless, these findings support the concept that population-focused approaches to reduce intake of sugar-sweetened beverages, such as changes in school or public policy, could be beneficial[123-126]. Dietary salt intake is associated with increased intake of sugar-sweetened beverages, perhaps because of increased thirst[127,128].

It is speculated that if the relationship is causal, it is possible that salt-reduction strategies could help to reduce intake of sugar-sweetened beverages.

Drugs and weight gain

A number of drugs can cause weight gain, including certain psychoactive drugs, antiepileptic drugs, and glucocorticoids[129,130]. Brief courses of oral or inhaled glucocorticoids are unlikely to have long-term effects on body weight unless they are prescribed frequently.

Weight gain and hyperlipidaemia are induced by psychoactive drugs, and some antidiabetic drugs are also known to cause weight gain[130].

The effects of SSRIs on body weight are less well characterised[131]. Although short-term use of some drugs have been associated with weight loss, long-term use of some SSRIs may be associated with weight gain[132].

PREVALENCE OF OVERWEIGHT AND OBESITY

Currently, almost one third of children and adolescents in the United States are either overweight or obese[133]. The population is distributed into higher weight categories with advancing age:

OVERWEIGHT OR OBESE

26.7% of preschool children (2 to 5 years)
32.6% of school-aged children (6 to 11 years)
33.6% of adolescents (12 to 19 years)

OBESE

12.1% of preschool children
18.0% of school-aged children
18.4% of adolescents

SEVERELY OBESE

9.7% of preschool children
13.0% of school-aged children
13.0% of adolescents

Severe obesity is thus present in 4.7% of children 6 to 11 years, and 6.3% of adolescents 12 to 17 years[134,135].

The prevalence of obesity is higher among Mexican Americans, non-Hispanic blacks, and American Indians than in non-Hispanic whites[13,133,134,136-138]. If a parent is obese it increases the risk by two- to threefold for a child to also develop obesity.

From a socioeconomic point of view, obesity is also more prevalent among low-income populations[139]. In 2010, 14.9% low-income children in the preschool age were obese (2.1% had extreme obesity) compared with 12.1% in the same age group from the general population[138].

The prevalence overweight and obesity in children is also increasing in most other developed countries worldwide. It is difficult to directly compare prevalence rates between countries because of differences in definitions and dates of measurements.

Use of the International Obesity Task Force (IOTF) standards typically results in lower prevalence estimates than other standards[140,141].

However, studies using comparable statistics show that rates are particularly high (greater than 30%) in most countries in North and South America, as well as in Great Britain, Greece, Italy, Malta, Portugal, and Spain[142]. There are somewhat lower rates in the Nordic countries, and the central portion of Western Europe.

In Russia and most of the countries of Eastern Europe the prevalence of overweight is lower (less than 10%), but increasing. In China, the prevalence of overweight among children is approximately 1/3 of that in the US, but a greater proportion of pre-school-aged children are affected[141].

Thus, across a wide range of developed and developing countries, and using a variety of measures, studies show increasing prevalence of obesity in children.

The increased prevalence of childhood obesity has resulted in an increased prevalence of the comorbidities associated with obesity[13]. As an example, the prevalence of conditions such as sleep apnoea and gall bladder disease in US children and adolescents tripled between 1979 and 1999[143].

Obesity trends

In the United States between 1976-2010 the prevalence of obesity among children (aged 6 to 11 years) and adolescents (aged 12 to 19 years) dramatically increased from 6.5% to 18.0% in children, and from 5.0% to 18.4% in adolescents[10,133].

During the same period the prevalence of obesity also doubled for younger children (aged 2 to 5 years) from 5% to 12.1%, where the increase in obesity prevalence reached a plateau around 2000 after which children and adolescents remained stable between 2000 and 2010[133].

Although obesity declined overall in girls in some states in the US between 2001 and 2008, it continued to increase for Black American girls[144].

In the United States the prevalence of obesity in children aged 2-5 years from low-income families has declined slightly in almost half of the states and is stable in the other half, but has increased in 3 states.

The slight decreases in childhood obesity have been reported in a few studies[145,146], whereas a few other studies have reported a plateau in the prevalence of childhood obesity[147,148].

From child to adolescent to adult

It is very difficult to predict which, or if, overweight children will end up obese when they become adults. The likelihood of persistence of childhood obesity into adulthood is to a large extent related to age[149-]

[151], if the parents are obese[34,152], and the severity of the obesity[153].

Observational studies have revealed that about 25% of obese preschool children remain obese when they become adults[154], compared to about 50% of obese 6-year-olds, and as many as 80% of obese 10 to 14-year-olds with at least one obese parent[34].

Another large cohort study reported that as many as 82% of children who were obese at age 11 years remained obese through adulthood during a follow up after 23 years[155].

It is also important to note that eating habits and levels of exercise often differ significantly between children in various studies. This may thus influence the predictability of the obesity risk in adulthood[19].

Not surprisingly, as a general rule an obese child with a sedentary lifestyle who does not change the caloric intake and lifestyle is unlikely to be of normal weight as an adult.

The severity of obesity through childhood, which continues during adolescence is an important predictor of whether the obesity will persist into adulthood, and thus how severe it will be[156].

This was confirmed in a study revealing that as many as 75% of adolescents in the United States with severe obesity (BMI >40) remained severely obese as adults[35], whereas only 8% of adolescents with moderate obesity will develop severe obesity as adults[156].

Whether gender influences the risk of obesity persisting into adulthood has been widely discussed and the results vary markedly between studies in different populations. As many as 80% of obese adolescent girls has been reported to remain obese into adulthood, whereas considerably fewer obese adolescent boys, i.e. 30% remained obese[157].

It is speculated that this gender difference is related to the differences and changes in puberty, when body fat decreases in boys as opposed to that in girls, where fat increases[158]. This is, however, in conflict with other studies presenting obesity in adolescent boys to be more likely to persist, and to be similar to that of girls[159-161].

There also seems to be geographic differences since a study from Australia reported that both boys and girls who were obese during adolescence had a 50 to 60% chance of remaining overweight as a young adult, not favouring one group from the other[161].

Interestingly, the same study noted that among adolescents who were not obese but merely overweight during adolescence, boys were actually slightly more likely than girls to remain obese during young adulthood[161].

The fact that socioeconomic differences are an issue in most health-related problems worldwide is well known. Obesity is, unfortunately, no exception. Obesity is considerably more common in most lower socioeconomic groups[162].

Although the exact reason for this is not clear, the cause is probably related to many different factors including education and understanding about food and nutrition as well as the benefits of exercise etc.[163,164].

Ethnicity is also an important factor known to influence obesity. Black men are reported to be less obese than white men whereas black women of all ages are more obese than white women[14]. The prevalence of obesity in Hispanic men and women is also reported to be higher than in white men and women[14].

The onset of obesity in young adulthood complicates the condition since it comes earlier and is faster in both black and Hispanic women than in white women[165].

NOTES

CAUSES OF OBESITY

Obesity can develop through a number of different causes. The most commonly discussed reasons for developing overweight and obesity are poor diet and lack of physical activity. The overall and fundamental cause of obesity is a chronic energy imbalance.

An energy intake that is higher than the energy expenditure over time inevitably leads to overweight, and if the energy intake is much higher than the energy expenditure the result will be obesity.

Several other causes may contribute to the development of obesity and must be taken into account, such as genetic predisposition and a number of underlying physical and psychological conditions. It is therefore crucial to include all aspects and causes of obesity to understand how obesity and its consequences can be effectively managed.

Several studies suggest that environmental and irregular eating habits that occur during critical periods in life may have permanent effects on obesity development and other metabolic diseases. However, specifically what drives people to eat unhealthy food is not clearly understood.

Although the actions of several appetite regulating hormones are known to influence hunger, the exact mechanisms are not yet fully explored or understood. In addition to the complicated physiology of appetite regulation, there are several environmental issues that influence appetite. The environmental influencers also need to be taken into account in the assessment of obesity.

Compared to that of hunger, there is considerably better understanding of satiety and discontinuing the eating process.

Distension of the gastrointestinal tract stimulates the release of hormones that send signals to the hypothalamus of the brain, which in turn promotes the feeling of satiety[166,167].

As mentioned, many things contribute to obesity. As many as 50 genetic factors are closely linked with obesity, BMI being the most well-known[168]. Other known causes of obesity include genetic diseases or brain injury caused by trauma, which in turn may influence appetite regulation[169].

Therefore, the cause of weight gain must always be thoroughly examined since an underlying disease may cause the obesity. Medication used in the treatment of such diseases and conditions can, subsequently, also stimulate and cause weight gain.

The rapid progression of obesity during the recent decades suggests that the environmental factors, such as the increase of fast food availability, are to a large extent driving the development of the disease. The genetic factors, however, are believed to determine if subjects are more or less predisposed to develop obesity[170].

Several practical, psychological and societal factors have been identified as contributing to energy imbalance. Food and beverages containing high calorie levels are cheap and widely available, and portion sizes have also increased.

Along with increased fat and sugar content in food and drinks, lifestyle also contributes to the energy imbalance. Physical activity has been significantly reduced due to new technologies that do not stimulate physical activity. Cellular phones are used instead of face-to-face contact. Spending more time at work may limit the time available for exercise and cooking, resulting in eating more processed and fast food[171,172].

Stress and fatigue can also influence exercise participation and eating habits. Other factors that have been implicated in energy imbalance include sleep disturbance, high consumption of transfats, infectious agents, perinatal exposure, and macronutrient quality[170].

Excess weight around the abdomen is specifically associated with greater risk of developing related disease such as cardiovascular problems and cancers[173].

Nutrition during pregnancy is thought to be an important determinant of metabolic programming, for example, a mother's body weight during pregnancy may influence body size, shape, and the subsequent body composition of the baby[174].

High pre-pregnancy BMI and excessive weight gain during pregnancy are also risk factors related to birth weight and childhood obesity[23].

In addition, infants born by diabetic mothers have a higher risk of becoming overweight as children, adolescents and adults[175,176]. The same applies to children born by mothers who smoked during pregnancy[177].

The prognostic value of childhood obesity is closely related to the age, onset and family history of the obesity[178]. Adolescent obesity is established before five years of age and is strongly associated with severe obesity in adulthood[35].

In addition to obesity, weight status in adolescence is important to predict later adverse health related problems[36]. Even though childhood and adolescent weight are of vital importance, most people suffering from overweight or obesity develop it during their adult life[176].

Most women suffering from overweight or obesity gain their excess weight after entering puberty[159]. Weight gain during pregnancy, and the effect of pregnancy on weight gain, are important in the weight gain history of women[179].

Although it may vary according to race and ethnic background, women usually increase their body weight and fat distribution slightly after their first pregnancy[180,181].

However, when compared with women who have not given birth, the overall risk of weight gain associated with pregnancy is probably limited in American women[182]. Weight gain is also associated with both oral contraceptives and menopause.

Weight gain and changes in fat distribution often occur during the early part of being postmenopausal[183]. However, the method used may significantly influence the outcome of the measurements[181]. One way of measuring is the bioelectrical impedence waist circumference measure[184].

Young men in their teens and twenties often lead a more active life. However, the level of activity decreases over time, towards a more sedentary lifestyle, often leading to weight gain. The weight gain often continues until the sixth decade before it stabilises, and thereafter starts to decline[176].

An increase in both visceral and non-visceral, specifically subcutaneous, body fat requires that energy intake be increased over energy expenditure.

However, other modulators are also important to take into account, such as intrauterine growth, growth hormone and reproductive hormone secretion, and the feedback between energy intake and expenditure[185].

The importance of the feedback control system has been associated with weight loss of as much 10 to 20% due to a decrease in total and resting energy expenditure, which slowed down further weight loss[186].

Weight gain is also associated with increased energy expenditure, which in turn should lead to slowed weight gain[187]. This is interesting since it suggests a mechanism that maintains body weight and therefore implies that other factors than behaviour influence obesity.

As a consequence, the changes in energy expenditure mean that someone who has previously been obese needs fewer calories to maintain normal body composition compared to someone with the same body composition who has not previously been obese.

Low energy expenditure is an important factor that can induce weight gain[188]. As much as 70% of energy expenditure is used for basal or resting metabolic processes, including maintaining body temperature, cardiac and respiratory function, gastrointestinal motility and secretion, and other naturally occurring energy consuming processes[189].

Brown adipose tissue (BAT) is known to regulate energy expenditure in infants and makes up about 5% of their body weight[190]. Through a specific heat-regulating process in BAT mitochondria generate heat instead of ATP which maintains normal body temperature[191].

BAT activity increases through childhood into adolescence up until around the age of 13 years in both boys and girls[192]. Thereafter, BAT decreases with age but is still metabolically active in adults[193-195]. BAT may be an important component of cold-stimulated energy expenditure in adults[196].

Anatomically, BAT is mostly located in the neck area and its activity is closely related to BMI and percent body fat[193,194].

Visceral fat is metabolically and hormonally more active than subcutaneous fat[197] and can result in an increased concentration of free fatty acids circulating in the blood leading to an increase of secreted adipokines, which in turn is linked to increased risk of heart disease[198].

Heart disease, hypertension, peripheral arterial disease, stroke, type 2 diabetes, gallbladder disease, osteoarthritis, and cancer, as well as insulin resistance, hyperinsulinaemia, and hyperlipidaemia, are all well known to be specifically associated with the excess of visceral fat.

Specific determination of fat deposition in people with lower BMI levels may be valuable in determining the prognosis of heart failure, since normal weight people with metabolic syndrome have increased heart failure risk compared with obese but healthy metabolic individuals[199].

Poor diet

Obesity is no doubt often the result of an excess of calorie intake. In nutritional contexts, the kilojoule (kJ) is used internationally for food energy. However, the calorie and kilocalorie are the most commonly used[200].

The average physically active man needs about 2,500 calories a day to maintain a normal and healthy weight, whereas the average physically active woman needs about 2,000 calories a day.

Obesity does not happen overnight – if it did, it could probably also be cured overnight. Obesity develops gradually over time as a result of poor diet, little or no physical activity, and other bad lifestyle choices.

Unhealthy eating habits are often seen in entire families since bad eating habits, including a diet high in fat and sugar, are often inherited from parents to children.

It is, therefore, not surprising that increased consumption of potato chips, potatoes, sugar-sweetened beverages, unprocessed red meat, and processed meats is directly associated with weight gain and subsequent obesity[117], and that a healthy diet of vegetables, whole grains, fruits, nuts, and yogurt has an opposite effect on weight gain and obesity.

Although high fat consumption has been pointed out as the cause of obesity for decades, lots of recent research suggest that sugar-sweetened beverages and fruit juices are directly related to the development of obesity in some individuals[201].

It is, however, important to point out that the effects of high consumptions of saturated fat on obesity are also significantly accentuated in individuals with specific genetic predispositions[202].

More recent evidence reveals that the combination of high consumption of sugar-sweetened beverages and a genetic predisposition seems to be a very important cause in the development of obesity[118,119].

No matter how we characterise the food intake, over-eating relative to energy expenditure will uniformly cause obesity since most obese people have lost control of their eating[110].

People who have normal weight often have a pattern of conscious limitations related to food intake, known as restrained eating[109]. This is more common in middle-aged women than in others.

Over or under-eating with respect to the frequency of meals and the development of obesity has been debated. Eating five meals daily instead of three has been presented to significantly lower the risk of overweight and obesity in adults[112] and in children[113].

One explanation for the effects of frequent small meals versus a few large meals could be the difference in insulin secretion associated with these meal sizes (that is increased with large meals)[203]. Although it is currently being debated, eating breakfast is associated with lower risk of overweight compared with people who skip it[114,204].

Binge-eating disorder, however, is a psychiatric illness characterised by uncontrolled episodes of eating that usually occur in the evening[205].

Lack of physical activity

Lack of physical activity is another important factor related to obesity. When people are not physically active, many consumed calories will be stored in the body as fat.

Jobs that involve sitting at a desk for most of the day without moving around are increasingly more common. People also rely more on cars as transportation instead of walking or cycling.

When people relax, they tend to watch TV, browse the Internet or play computer games, and rarely do regular exercise. Unfortunately, the same goes for children. Physical activity is important to burn off the energy provided by the consumed food to ensure that it is not stored as fat.

Many different recommendations about how much time should be used weekly for physical activity have been presented. The WHO recommends adults do at least 150 minutes of moderate-intensity aerobic activity, such as cycling or fast walking, every week[206].

The exercise does not need to be carried out all at once. Divided into smaller sessions, for example, 30 minutes a day for five days will work just as well, or even better.

Obese people attempting to lose weight might require more exercise than 150 minutes weekly. Obesity is inversely related to moderately vigorous physical activity, totally in contrast to the opposite, a sedentary lifestyle[207].

It appears that the effects of TV on obesity are not solely related to changes in physical activity alone but is also facilitated by changes in energy intake[208,209].

Lack of, or irregular, sleep is also suggested to lead to obesity[82,210]. Also, lack of sleep may possibly reduce the proportion of weight lost during caloric restriction[211]. This can probably be partly explained by the influence that sleep has on different hormones that stimulate hunger and appetite[212-214].

Genetics

Genetic factors are important and interact closely with environmental factors in the development of obesity. Genetic factors account for as much as 30 to 50% of the cause of obesity[215].
A variety of specific syndromes and gene defects linked to childhood obesity are well known. These are rare causes of obesity, accounting for less than 1% of childhood obesity in specialist (tertiary) care centres[10,216,217].

In addition to being overweight, children with obesity-related genetic syndromes typically have findings on physical examination, e.g. dysmorphic features, short stature, developmental delay or intellectual disability (mental retardation), retinal changes, or deafness.

For most syndromes the genetic cause has been identified to enable specific testing and examination, but exactly how they cause obesity is not entirely understood.

Although it is still rare (about 4-6%), mutations in the melanocortin 4 receptor is the most common single gene defect in people suffering from severe obesity[218,219].

The effects of microbes, infections and toxins on obesity

The human gut harbours a complex community of microbes that may affect many aspects of our health. Recent studies have suggested that different types of gut microbes are closely linked to obesity[220] and its treatment[221,222].

The gut microbes do not only play an important role in the development of obesity and obesity-associated inflammation, but they also affect insulin resistance[223]. Genetics influence the structure of the human gut microbes and may therefore influence metabolism differently[224].

It is also possible that obesity can be triggered or worsened by a virus, especially the adenovirus 36 which increases body fat in animals[225], and in both children and adults there is an association between adenovirus 36 and obesity[221].

Several studies have presented the relationship between weight gain and resistant bacteria[226-231]. Another hypothesis is that different types of resident bacteria mixed together have a greater potential of saving calories from fermentation[232]

Exposure to environmental endocrine disrupting chemicals, such as bisphenol A (BPA), used for packaging of food, are believed to be a part of the cause of obesity[233].

BPA can be detected in urine and most of the exposure is believed to come from food[234]. Studies demonstrate an association between urinary BPA concentrations and obesity or obesity-related diseases, including diabetes and cardiovascular disease in both adults and children[235-238].

In addition, BPA is a selective modulator of oestrogen receptors, and is therefore thought to accelerate adipogenesis and postnatal growth[239-241].

Genetic factors have been clearly established in obesity studies of twins, adoptees, and families[242,243]. In twins the heritability of obesity is high with only slightly lower values in twin raised apart compared with those raised together[244].

Similarly, in adoptees the body mass index correlates with that of their biologic parents rather than that of their adoptive parents[245].

In addition to the heredity related to overweight and obesity, metabolic rate, thermic response to food, and spontaneous physical activity are also to a certain extent related to heredity[243]. This suggests that both current weight status, including weight gain, and the metabolic processes are closely related to heredity.

Obesity is also closely related to as many as 24 genetic disorders[246]. The Prader-Willi[247] and Bardet-Biedl[248] syndromes are probably the best known examples of genetic disorders leading to obesity.

The Prader-Willi syndrome is a neurodegenerative disorder caused by abnormalities of chromosome 15 where the majority of patients have a deletion of paternal DNA and a few have two copies of maternal chromosome 15.

The chromosome usually lacks a gene that codes for a ribonucleoprotein, which is believed to be involved in imprinting genes from both parents[249,250].

Infants with Prader-Willi syndrome have poor muscle tone and tend to not feed well at birth and shortly thereafter. The hunger and appetite, however, subsequently increases considerably which leads to obesity[251]. Other symptoms and signs include delayed development, short stature, behaviour problems such as irritability and tantrums, followed by hypogonadotropic hypogonadism.

If Prader-Willi syndrome is identified and treated early, the prognosis is good and patients can lead relatively normal lives[252]. Although the condition is very rare and data in significant numbers are unavailable in adult patients, spontaneous menarche, followed by irregular menses, and amenorrhea have been presented[251].

The Bardet-Biedl syndrome is characterised by obesity, mental retardation, and several other abnormalities including cilia dysfunction[253,254]. Mutations in at least 15 genes are present in patients with this Bardet-Biedl syndrome[255].

Obesity is thus, unquestionably an inherited condition in these complex genetic disorders, but the genes that contribute to the more common forms of obesity have been difficult to identify. Many studies in large populations have, however, been able to identify a number of specific genes that are associated with increased risk of more common types of obesity, further confirming its genetic importance[256-263].

A variant in the fat mass and obesity associated (FTO) gene on chromosome 16 is known to increase the risk of developing type 2 diabetes[257].

Also, this variant also increases the risk of developing overweight and thus obesity in the general population, where a significant increased risk of obesity is seen in both adults and children[257,264]. The FTO is suggested to be responsible for as much as 22 percent of obesity[264].

Brain-derived neurotrophic factor (BDNF) may play a role in energy balance and associated with childhood-onset obesity[265,266]. The BDNF is associated with a 10% increased risk of developing obesity[267]. However, this has not been confirmed in all populations[268].

Retinaldehyde is an interesting intermediate metabolite that is showing promise in suppressing adipogenesis. Increasing retinaldehyde in fat protects against obesity and insulin resistance[269]. However, the effects of retinaldehyde need to be further explored.

Hormones and appetite control

The appetite regulating hormones in the gut are probably the most important factors in the regulation of obesity and are therefore interesting in the development of new obesity and diabetes therapies[270].

Simply put, the regulation of appetite is the feeling of hunger when you need to eat, and the feeling of being full when you need to stop eating, but the exact physiology of how the appetite is regulated is complicated[271,272].

Appetite is important in the process of gaining and losing weight and is influenced by a number of different mechanisms to keep a stable body weight. A calorie increase of as little as 0.5% over the energy expenditure is enough to cause weight gain[273].

The hypothalamus in the brain is fundamental in regulating appetite[274], especially since gut hormone receptors are located in the hypothalamus[275].

Gut hormone receptors in the brain thus play an important role in the response to signals from circulating hormones influencing appetite and obesity[276]. This signalling is known as the gut-brain axis.

A number of appetite regulating hormones have been mentioned as being involved in appetite regulation. Signals from leptin and insulin are associated with upholding both short and long-term energy balance, whereas ghrelin, peptide YY, pancreatic polypeptide, glucagon-like peptide-1 (GLP-1) and oxyntomodulin are influenced and controlled by eating[272].

Leptin is a hormone produced by fat cells and it regulates the amount of fat stored in the body[277]. It is referred to as the satiety hormone (the sensation of being full after eating) since it affects both the sensation of hunger, and the energy expenditures[278].

Although leptin reduces appetite as a circulating signal, obese individuals generally exhibit a higher circulating concentration of leptin than normal weight individuals due to their higher percentage body fat[279].

Although not as efficient as leptin, insulin is also believed to have influence appetite[280]. Also, insulin resistance is believed to increase obesity[281,282].

Ghrelin is one of the gastrointestinal hormones produced mostly in the stomach[283], and is the only known appetite stimulating hormone[284]. Not surprisingly, ghrelin is also known as the hunger hormone. The secretion starts when the stomach is empty and stops when the stomach is stretched[285].

Interestingly, ghrelin stimulates appetite in the same way in both lean and obese people[286,287]. Ghrelin levels are negatively correlated with weight, i.e. in obese people the levels are lower than in leaner individuals, indicating that ghrelin does not cause obesity[288].

The ghrelin receptor is located in the hypothalamus on the same cells where the leptin receptors are found, i.e. both the hunger and satiety hormone receptors are located beside each other in the brain[289].

Glucagon-like peptide 1 (GLP-1) is another gut hormone released by the intestinal L cells primarily in the small intestine[290], which increases insulin and decreases glucagon secretion from the pancreas. GLP-1 is currently used as an effective treatment of type 2 diabetes[291].

The secretion of GLP-1 is dependent on ingestion of food and is therefore an important appetite regulating hormone since it decreases food intake by increasing satiety[292].

The effects of GLP-1 on regulating food intake are probably also regulated by other functions since the GLP-1 levels have been reported to rise prior to eating, i.e. in the anticipation of having a meal[293].

Another effect of GLP-1, besides reducing food intake, is that it supresses secretion of glucagon, which in turn delays gastric emptying[294], and the reduced food intake affects both obese and normal weight people[295].

Cholesytokinin (CCK) is a peptide hormone in the gut responsible for stimulating the digestion of protein and fat, and for more than four decades it has been known to be involved in appetite control [296].

It is synthesised and released widely throughout the gastrointestinal tract, but mostly in the jejunum and duodenum[297], and in the hypothalamus[298].

CCK has a number of physiological effects including the stimulation of gallbladder contraction and pancreatic and gastric acid secretion, slowing of gastric emptying and suppression of energy intake[299].

Pancreatic polypeptide (PP) is a peptide hormone that is mostly secreted from cells in the Islets of Langerhans-part of the pancreas[276]. The PP levels are reduced with increased food intake and elevated during hunger[300]. In addition, PP reduces appetite and leads to decreased food intake, leading to reduction of body weight[300-302].

Peptide YY (PPY), also known as peptide tyrosine tyrosine or pancreatic peptide YY, is an appetite reducing peptide hormone released in the ileum and colon in response to food intake[303]. The development of obesity may be partly influenced by the hormone, since the secretion of PPY is usually lower in obese people[304,305].

However, leptin is also known to reduce appetite in response to food intake, but obese people develop a resistance to leptin indicating that reduction in PYY sensitivity probably only plays a minimal role in the cause of obesity. This is also in contrast to the reduction of leptin sensitivity which plays a more important role in the development of obesity[306].

High appetite reducing effects of PPY is seen in both lean and obese people, where as much as a 30% calorie decrease is reported[307].

Oxyntomodulin (OXM) is a peptide hormone secreted from L cells in the jejunum, ileum and colon, following food intake[308,309]. It binds to both the GLP-1 and the glucagon receptor[310,311].

Other important functions of OXM is inhibiting gastric acid secretion and delaying of gastric emptying, which thereby decreases food intake[312,313]. Besides the decrease in food intake, OXM also causes weight loss through increased energy expenditure[314].

Although its action is not as powerful, OXM reveal incretin, i.e. gut hormones stimulate a decrease in blood glucose levels, functions similar to those of GLP-1[315], suggesting that GLP-1 is more effective in type 2 diabetes treatment. However, a study revealed that weight loss was superior in mice given OXM compared with GLP-1[316].

There are a few other less well-understood peptides that may influence appetite and obesity. Bombesin is present in the gastrointestinal tract and acts by supressing food intake[317,318]. Amylin is released by the pancreas and decreases gastric emptying and reduces food intake by increasing satiety[319,320].

Finally, fibroblast growth factors (FGFs) are metabolic regulators that affect insulin sensitivity and lipid metabolism[321]. Perhaps more important, also increases leptin sensitivity[322].

Although it is rare, excessive weight gain may be a symptom of another disease. Medical causes of obesity can include hypothyroidism, a condition where the thyroid gland does not produce enough thyroid hormone[323]. Thyroid hormone regulates metabolism, specifically by increasing the overall rate of energy metabolism[324].

Hypothyroidism therefore slows the metabolism which subsequently leads to weight gain. Other conditions include Cushing's syndrome and depression. Cushing's syndrome is a condition which occurs when the adrenal glands produce an excess amount of cortisol[325]. This leads to a build-up of fat in the face, upper back, and abdomen. Depression often leads to overeating, which will inevitably lead to obesity[326].

Endocrine causes are present in very few children and adolescents suffering from obesity[217], and those causes identified are usually only associated with overweight or mild obesity rather than severe obesity[216].

However, acquired hypothalamic conditions and injuries may lead to severe obesity, and are very difficult to treat. The most commonly diagnosed acquired hypothalamic problems are neural crest tumours identified in children, which leads to short stature and/or hypogonadism[217].

Obesity has many other causes related to diseases and disorders of the brain, each of which may be inherited[185,327,328]. One type of obesity may be caused by single-gene mutations[329], whereas various diseases or injuries to the brain in people in whom obesity would otherwise not occur may cause another type[185].

Also, drug-induced obesity, or iatrogenic obesity, is a condition where various types of drugs, e.g. steroids, antidepressants, high blood pressure drugs, and seizure medications also lead to obesity[330].

DISEASES, CONDITIONS AND DISORDERS INFLUENCED BY OBESITY

Both the environment and nutrition are important influencers during critical periods in childhood development and may affect the risk of developing obesity and metabolic disease. The exact causes and mechanisms have not been specifically established, and are therefore being investigated[331].

The endocrine profile and eating habits during pregnancy is an important predictor of metabolic programming (intrauterine development that may subsequently determine the health and disease later in life). Babies born small for gestational age (SGA), or those born large for gestational age (LGA) often have higher rates of insulin resistance during childhood and adolescence[332-334].

An association between birth weight and subsequent diabetes, heart disease, insulin resistance, and obesity is also well known[335,336]. Several studies have confirmed the causal links between exposures to various types and amounts of food during pregnancy and subsequent obesity and metabolic disease[337-339].

A mother's weight prior to her pregnancy and her weight gain during the pregnancy are essential to the birth weight of the child, including all additional environmental factors related to pregnancy[334,340,341].

Gestational diabetes is associated with subsequent increased BMI in both boys and adult males, independent of the mother's BMI during early pregnancy[342].

Maternal preeclampsia is also related to higher BMI when the child reaches adolescence[343,344]. This has been reported to be present in both boys[344,345] and girls[346].

Women who have had gastric bypass surgery appear to give birth to children with a lower prevalence of obesity than children born before the mother has had gastric bypass. This indicates that reversal of maternal obesity leads to beneficial permanent effects on the metabolic profile of the child[347].

The newborn period and early childhood are also important periods for the metabolic programming. There are clear associations between weight gain during early life and the subsequent obesity or metabolic syndrome in early childhood[348-350], and in both adolescence and adulthood[351].

This has also been reported in systematic reviews[352-355], and in other early childhood-related conditions, e.g. blood pressure and other cardiovascular risk factors[356-359]. Together with metabolic programming, this evidence strongly indicates that early intervention is an important tool in preventing obesity.

Also, there's a lot of data supporting efforts to improve and optimise eating habits in pregnant women, newborns and young children. Such improvements especially include optimising glycaemic control in pregnant women and targeting weight gain in newborns and young children.

The subsequent growth in newborns with low birth weight improves the outcome of neural development, but at the same time it is also associated with increased risks for various metabolic complications[360-363].

Increasing the protein content of our food appears to lower and thus normalise IGF-1 concentrations[360]. Although it needs to be further explored, this has been suggested to further improve neural development and metabolic stability for infants.

The age, especially in younger mothers, is an important predictor of the child's subsequent obesity status, and besides obesity status it is also closely related to socioeconomic factors[364].

Without distinguishing between mechanisms of metabolic programming versus genetic obesity factors during pregnancy, mothers who had early menarche have children with accelerated growth during the first years of life, after which time the growth rate normalises. [365].

Maternal BMI appears to be a more reliable predictor for obesity development than metabolic programming with respect to intergenerational transmission of obesity.

Psychological aspects of obesity

Although depression is hard to predict based on different personality types, psychological issues are important in the development of obesity. People with severe obesity often suffer from depression[366]. Also, patients tend to gain weight easier during wintertime indicating a causal relationship between the cold and (or) dark season and weight gain and obesity[367].

Endocrine effects of obesity

Obesity has become one of the most important public health problems, especially in the United States[10-12]. It is well known that as the prevalence of obesity increases so does the prevalence of the comorbidities associated with obesity[13].

For this reason it is absolutely essential that health care providers learn to both predict and identify unhealthy weight gain, overweight and obesity in children so that counselling and treatment can be provided.

The consequences of obesity in childhood and adolescence include abnormalities in the endocrine, cardiovascular, gastrointestinal, pulmonary, orthopaedic, neurologic, dermatologic and psychosocial systems[368].

Some conditions that used to be considered adult diseases are now regularly seen in children suffering from obesity, for example, type 2 diabetes. Needless to say, the earlier onset, and the longer people suffer from such conditions the more severe the consequences.

Obesity during adolescence increases the risk for developing related diseases and premature death during adulthood, independent of the severity of obesity during adulthood[36,369-371].

For example, women who were overweight during childhood have an increased risk of developing breast cancer, with a subsequent increased mortality risk in adulthood[36].

Likewise, men who were overweight during childhood have a higher risk of developing ischemic heart disease and subsequently are at higher risk of dying from it as adults.

Endocrine conditions caused by obesity in children and adolescents include impaired glucose tolerance, diabetes mellitus, and different abnormalities in growth and puberty.

Impaired glucose tolerance and obesity

Impaired glucose tolerance is a good predictor of diabetes and is a common complication associated with both childhood and adolescent obesity[372,373].

The reported prevalence of impaired glucose tolerance and type 2 diabetes in obese children vary considerably, probably because of differences in degree of obesity between children, geographic and ethnic variation, and age range of the sampled population.

Studying sixth graders revealed that 30% were overweight and over 20% of obese children, and almost 23% of severely obese children had impaired glucose tolerance[374,375].

Another study of obese children and adolescents revealed that 25% of children and 21% of adolescents had evidence of impaired glucose tolerance, measured by oral glucose tolerance tests[376].

The prevalence of impaired glucose tolerance in obese children and adolescents ranges from 7 to 13.5%, and the prevalence of type 2 diabetes was between 1-2%[377-379].

Because insulin resistance, together with BMI, is a good predictor of impaired glucose tolerance, it is probably also useful to measure insulin resistance in overweight and obese children and adolescents, but there is not yet consensus about the test accuracy for insulin resistance in children.

The euglycemic clamp is considered to be the standard method in research, but it is considered to be too invasive for patients in clinical practice[380].

Insulin resistance is when the body produces insulin, but the cells in the body become resistant to insulin and are unable to use it effectively, leading to hyperglycaemia[381]. There are several surrogate measures for insulin resistance.

The three most commonly used are the homeostasis model assessment of insulin resistance (HOMA)[382], the fasting glucose-to-insulin ratio (FGIR)[383-385], and the quantitative insulin sensitivity check index (QUICKI)[386]. However, the validity of surrogate measures for insulin resistance have been reported to have limitations[387].

In obese children and adolescents insulin resistance have been assessed using different confirmatory tests (oral glucose tolerance test, frequent sampling intravenous glucose tolerance test, and clamp testing) resulting in different outcomes[380,388-392]. Other ways of measuring insulin sensitivity come from collecting data from oral glucose tolerance tests[393].

Impaired glucose tolerance and insulin resistance, in obese children and adolescents, are usually measured by evaluating fasting glucose and/or measuring Haemoglobin A_{1c} (HbA$_{1c}$).

A fasting plasma glucose level of between 100 and 125 mg/dL, or a HbA_{1c} between 5.7% and 6.4%, indicates pre-diabetes with an increased risk of developing type 2 diabetes. This should, therefore, be further evaluated, and followed up with an oral glucose tolerance test[394].

Type 2 diabetes mellitus and obesity

Type 2 diabetes mellitus (T2DM) is a serious consequence of obesity in children and adolescents[395-397]. Early diagnosis and treatment is crucial to slow down the development of complications which include retinopathy, neuropathy, nephropathy, and cardiovascular problems[398].

Furthermore, people who were diagnosed with T2DM during adolescence have a faster progression of diabetes-related complications compared with those who receive the diagnosis later in life. Newly diagnosed T2DM in adolescent patients often reveal several related comorbidities.

A study revealed that 13.0% had microalbuminuria, 80.5% had dyslipidaemia, and 13.6% had hypertension[399]. Also, and not surprisingly, a study revealed a clear association between high BMI in adolescent men and T2DM during adulthood[400].

In the same study, it is important to note that the association actually disappeared after adjusting for BMI during adulthood. This suggests that T2DM is primarily associated with obesity around the time of the diagnosis, and not the effects of chronic obesity since childhood.

Another study revealed that people who were overweight or obese while they were children but who were not obese as adults had similar risk of developing T2DM compared with individuals who had not previously been obese[155].

Metabolic syndrome and obesity

The metabolic syndrome is a term used to describe the clustering of metabolic risk factors for type 2 diabetes and atherosclerotic cardiovascular disease in adults: abdominal obesity, hyperglycaemia, dyslipidaemia, and hypertension[401].

Several cardiovascular risks are also present in children and adolescents who are overweight and/or obese[402]. About 10% of US adolescents are reported to have metabolic syndrome according to the same criteria used for adults[403-405].

This is, however, not entirely reliable since puberty is associated with a number of changes related, or comparable to the metabolic syndrome.

About half of adolescents initially classified as having metabolic syndrome actually did not meet the criteria for the diagnosis at a three-year follow-up examination[406]. It is also worth noting that during the same period many subjects not initially diagnosed with metabolic syndrome acquired it.

Although a number of schemes have been developed to classify the metabolic syndrome in adolescents, the long-term consequences of the condition in children and adolescents are still not fully understood[407,408].

Puberty, growth and obesity

Obesity may lead to accelerated growth and bone age[409]. It remains unclear if the accelerated growth results in overweight and obesity which is different from the genetic programming.

Although the relationship is not entirely consistent[410], overweight is associated with early puberty in girls[411,412]. There is also inconsistency about the onset of puberty in boys[411,413].

Cardiovascular effects of obesity

Obesity in children and adolescents is associated with a number of cardiovascular changes that are linked to increased cardiovascular risk in adulthood[38]. Two of these, hypertension and dyslipidaemia, are components of the metabolic syndrome[414].

Only 4.2% of obese children and adolescents have no evidence of cardiovascular risk factors, i.e. so called metabolically healthy obesity, and tend to remain metabolically healthy in adulthood[415].

Hypertension and obesity

The risk of developing hypertension is considerably increased in overweight and obese children and adolescents[416]. Those who are obese have approximately three times higher risk of developing hypertension than children and adolescents who are only overweight[417].

When hypertension is diagnosed by using normal blood pressure monitoring in a hospital setting, as many as 50% of obese children have the condition[418,419]. However, when the blood pressure is measured in a casual office setting, fewer cases of hypertension are diagnosed[420].

This is called masked hypertension, and is particularly common in children with obesity, and may result in clinically important consequences[421].

Elevated BMI is also associated with increased left ventricular mass in children both with and without hypertension[416,422-426]. Childhood hypertension is a good predictor of adult hypertension and metabolic syndrome[427].

Obesity during childhood thus predicts hypertension during adulthood even if the individual loses weight by adulthood[155].

Dyslipidaemia and obesity

Dyslipidaemia is an abnormal amount of lipids in the blood and usually occurs among overweight and obese children and adolescents, especially individuals with a central fat distribution[428-432].

Typically the concentrations of serum LDL-cholesterol and triglycerides are elevated and the concentration of HDL-cholesterol is decreased[416,430-432].

Determining hyperlipidaemia in obese children and adolescents includes evaluating the measurement of a fasting lipid panel, including total cholesterol, triglycerides, and HDL-cholesterol.

Childhood obesity also leads to a number of other risk factors for developing atherosclerosis[419,433-442], suggesting that the development of atherosclerosis begins at an early age.

This also indicates that atherosclerosis is not only related to inflammation, hypertension, and abnormal lipid profiles, but it is also closely associated with obesity[443,444]. Insulin resistance is another independent risk factor for early onset of carotid atherosclerosis[445].

Cardiovascular risk factors are significantly elevated in young overweight people, but are even more serious in those who are obese, suggesting that even a minor excess of fat increases the risk of developing cardiovascular disease[446].

Adult coronary heart disease and obesity

The increasing evidence thus demonstrates a clear association between high BMI and obesity during childhood and the critical outcome of other cardiovascular events in adults [447].

BMI in 17 year old men is also closely associated with coronary heart disease during adulthood, and this association persists even after adjusting for adult BMI[400].

This clearly indicates that the underlying causes of coronary heart disease begins during adolescence. It is further confirmed by monitoring how changes in obesity status affect cardiovascular risk factors during adulthood[155].

It is estimated that by 2035, in the US alone, more than 100,000 additional cases of coronary heart disease will be caused by the increase in childhood obesity[448]. Also, ischaemic stroke is increased in both obese men and women[449].

Women with a BMI above 30 have 70% greater risk of developing stroke[450], while the risk of developing stroke in men with BMI above 30 is even higher, i.e. 100% greater compared to men with normal BMI[451].

Other cardiovascular and related conditions associated with obesity are migraines and headaches. Obesity is thought to be associated with episodic and chronic migraines where obesity is clearly an exacerbating factor[452]. Headaches are also significantly more common and severe in obese people than in normal weight people[453].

Gastrointestinal effects of obesity

Obesity is associated with several liver abnormalities jointly called non-alcoholic fatty liver disease (NAFLD)[216,454]. The NAFLD condition is the most common cause of liver disease in children[455,456].

Non-alcoholic fatty liver disease includes two different types: steatosis (increased liver fat without inflammation) and non-alcoholic steatohepatitis (increased liver fat with inflammation).

If it is not treated properly, non-alcoholic steatohepatitis may lead to fibrosis, cirrhosis, and ultimately liver failure[457]. Although the pathogenesis of NAFLD in overweight and obese individuals remains to be further explored insulin resistance is suggested to be closely associated[458,459].

Independent of the degree of obesity, the metabolic syndrome and NAFLD are also clinically associated through insulin resistance, dyslipidaemia, and hypertension[460]. The prevalence of NAFLD in children is increasing along with increased obesity[461-463].

The prevalence of fatty liver is as high as 38% in obese children compared to 9.6% in the overall population[464], and steatohepatitis is seen in 23% of subjects with fatty liver, amounting to about 3% of the general population [461]. Although the prevalence differs geographically it is consistently increased with obesity[465,466].

Most people with NAFLD initially rarely experience symptoms or signs of liver disease[216]. Those who do experience symptoms usually feel right upper quadrant pain or general abdominal discomfort, weakness, fatigue or malaise[467,468].

Imaging and laboratory tests reveal the abnormalities and confirm the presence of fatty liver[216,468-473], but the abnormalities resolve with weight loss[468,474].

The severity of the liver disease cannot be determined with radiographic features, clinical features, or the degree of elevation of liver transaminases[19,473,475,476].

Ultrasonography is frequently used to confirm the presence of fatty liver and other conditions such as the presence of splenomegaly and liver nodularity even though the clinical uncertainty in the diagnosis of fatty liver disease is debatable[477].

Liver biopsy is another, more reliable, diagnostic tool. Even so, the clinical value of the liver biopsy for suspected NAFLD needs to be further established in both children and adults. Therefore this examination also remains debatable[471].

Still, the liver biopsy is the only reliable test to distinguish simple steatosis, steatohepatitis, and fibrosis from one another.

Weight management is the only established treatment for NAFLD; small non-randomised studies in children have shown improvement after weight loss[468,471,478-480].

Emphasis on physical activity is appropriate because of its utility in improving insulin sensitivity, which appears to be an important pathway for the development of NAFLD.

Since most people with NAFLD are overweight or obese, and the only current treatment for NAFLD is weight management, the results of a liver biopsy are therefore not likely to provide any relevant information. If NAFLD is suspected, weight management should be initiates as soon as posssible.

People with early onset of NAFLD or other signs or symptoms suggesting significant serious liver problems should be evaluated for other conditions that look like fatty liver in young children[481]. In such cases more intensive tests are warranted.

Physical activity improves NAFLD independent of weight loss[482]. As the first-line treatment for obese children with NAFLD the American Gastroenterological Association suggest lifestyle changes aiming at weight loss[481].

The use of vitamin E, metformin and thiazolidinediones may be beneficial, but none of them are as effective as lifestyle interventions[483-485]. Any improvement is therefore most likely due to weight loss[481].

Obesity is the most common cause of gallstones in children without predisposing causes[486-488]. The risk of developing gallstones increases with BMI and is considerably greater for girls than boys, and can increase as much as sevenfold in severely obese girls compared with normal-weight girls[489].

The risk is further increased in girls using oral contraceptives, and ethnicity also influences the risk factor for developing gallstones[490].

Signs and symptoms of gallstones in children and adolescents are non-specific and are hard to detect[488,491,492]. The symptoms include epigastric and right upper quadrant pain, jaundice, nausea, vomiting, and fatty food intolerance[486,487,491].

Early detection is necessary for successful management. Gallbladder disease should always be considered in overweight or obese adolescents with persisting abdominal pain[216].

Gastroesophageal reflux disease is also more common in obese than in normal weight people[493].

Respiratory effects of obesity

Respiratory problems related to obesity in children and adolescents include obstructive sleep apnoea (OSA) and the obesity hypoventilation syndrome (OHS). OSA describes complete obstruction of the upper airway during sleep and cessation of air movement despite ongoing respiratory effort.

Partial airway obstruction is called obstructive hypoventilation. OSA is typically but not always associated with persistent snoring. The prevalence of OSA is higher in obese children and adolescents than in healthy weight subjects[494].

There are a number of issues that make the relationship between sleep and obesity rather complex. Shorter duration of sleep can lead to obesity[495]. Obstructive sleep apnoea is associated with decreased insulin sensitivity in adolescents, independent of obesity.

Patients with obesity also may have hypoventilation during sleep in the absence of airway obstruction, probably caused by the restrictive ventilatory defect in obese people, often with severe oxygen desaturation[494].

Obese children and adolescents with breathing problems caused by sleep disorders should be referred for specialty care[216,496].

These patients need an immediate and strict weight loss program since rapid weight loss, sometimes combined with continuous positive airway pressure treatment can significantly improve breathing[496].

Orthopaedic and rheumatologic effects of obesity

The profound damaging effects that obesity has on the locomotor system are well known and established. That osteoarthritis of the knee is associated with overweight and obesity has been known for decades[497].

People with a BMI greater than 26.4 have 6 times higher rate of knee osteoarthritis than subjects with a BMI less than 23.4[498]. Osteoarthritis in obese people is not only seen in the knee but also in other weight-bearing and non-weight-bearing joints[449].

Obesity and overweight also seriously affects rheumatoid arthritis and how well treatments works[499]. Apart from losing weight, regular physical activity before rheumatoid arthritis is diagnosed also positively affects the treatment outcome[500].

Men with a BMI of 30-35 have 2.3 times higher risk of gout, while a BMI of 35 and above increases the gout risk 3 times compared to that of people with normal BMI[501]. Lowering BMI thus decreases the risks of gout.

Other obesity-related problems of the locomotor system include slipped capital femoral epiphysis (SCFE) and tibia vara (or Blount disease).

Obese children also have an increased risk of fractures, genu valgum, impaired mobility, and general musculoskeletal pain (e.g. back, hip, leg, knee, ankle, and foot), compared with non-obese children[502-505].

Obesity is a significant risk factor in SCFE, which is characterised by a displacement of the capital femoral epiphysis from the femoral neck through the growth plate[506].

The condition, which is diagnosed through x-rays, often occurs in late childhood or early adolescence, and the patients often complain about dull, aching pain in the hip, groin, thigh, or knee, without preceding history of trauma. Once the diagnose is confirmed weight loss is crucial to prevent contralateral SCFE[496].

Tibia vara is characterised by disturbance of normal growth in the inner part of the upper tibia. Tibia vara causes a bowlegged gait and can impair the knees significantly[507]. It results from inhibited growth of the medial proximal tibial growth plate due to abnormal weight bearing of the knee[508,509].

Tibia vara is closely associated with obesity[507,509-514]. Other clinical features of the condition include complaints of knee pain or instability and bowlegs that gradually increase in severity[461,515].

Severe obesity may disguise the condition and thus delay the diagnosis. X-rays are necessary to establish the diagnosis. Tibia vara is reported to be more common in children of African ancestry[508,510,512,514].

Obese children are generally more susceptible to fractures than normal weight children[504]. Obese children generally have reduced bone mass, unlike adults[516-518].

The effects of stress from body weight during falls, vitamin D deficiency, reduced bone mass from lack of exercise, and other biomechanical effects of obesity on the skeleton needs to be further established[519].

Also, unspecific low back pain and several other musculoskeletal pains and disability problems are between 2-4 times as prevalent in obese people compared with normal weight people[520].

Cancer effects of obesity

In 2008, there were an estimated 12.7 million cancer cases and 7.6 million cancer deaths worldwide. This, despite the fact that many cancers are preventable[521,522].

Survival rates are improving, but over half a million people die from cancer each year in the US alone. Cancer outranks cardiovascular disease as the number one cause of death in the US for those under the age of 85[523].

Between 5% and as many as 20% of cancers are due to overweight and obesity[524,525]. As many as 17 out of 22 types of cancers are associated with elevated BMI, including breast and ovarian, oesophageal and colorectal, liver and pancreatic, gallbladder and stomach, endometrial and cervical, prostate and kidney, etc.[526,527]. The increased risk of developing cancer as a consequence of overweight and obesity is 9% and in postmenopausal breast cancer up to as much as 39% in endometrial cancer[528].

There is also a significant direct associations with additional cancers including pancreas, thyroid, non-Hodgkin lymphoma, leukaemia, and myeloma[529]. Emerging evidence suggests a role for obesity in aggressive prostate cancer[530]. Bariatric surgery reduces general cancer mortality with as much as 60%[531].

Gaining or reducing weight is also associated with an increased cancer risk. The risk of colorectal cancer increases with 60% in men who gain 21 kg or more after the age of 20 than men who only gain between 1 and 5 kg[532]. Also, women who lose 10 kg or more after menopause reduces the breast cancer risk with 50%[533].

The effects of obesity and weight change probably vary depending on tumour site with emphasis on endogenous oestrogens in breast and endometrial cancer and on insulin and inflammation in colon cancer[525].

Low levels of physical activity likely increase the risk for cancer[534]. Well over 60% of adults in the US do not exercise regularly, where over 25% are almost entirely sedentary[535]. Leading a sedentary lifestyle is believed to cause 5% of cancer deaths[536].

For people who do not smoke, together with weight control and a healthy diet, exercise is the most important preventive action against risk factors[537]. Exercise is known to decrease the risk of developing colon, liver, pancreas, and stomach cancer[538].

The strongest data connecting obesity and cancer come from colon and breast cancer[528,539-541]. Strenuous long-term exercise activity acts as a protector against invasive and in situ breast cancer[540].

More active individuals also have 24% reduced risk of developing colon cancer compared to those who are minimally active[528].

Similarly, when comparing the most and least physically active, the risk of developing both proximal and distal colorectal cancer is reduced by 27% in the more active individuals[542]. Physical activity also significantly affects the colon polyps, reducing the risk by 15%[543].

The protective effect of activity goes beyond its impact on body weight since the association between physical activity and decreased risk of developing breast or colon cancer is seen across all levels of obesity[538,544-546].

Although the data is not as comprehensive as for breast and colorectal cancers, physical activity also protects against endometrial and prostate cancer[528,547,548].

There are many protective mechanisms contributing to the effects of physical activity include reduction of circulating hormones (such as insulin) and other growth factors, altered prostaglandin levels, altered bile acid metabolism and generally improved immune function[549-551].

Physical activity during adolescence also offers protection against diseases including breast cancer[552,553], but the optimal duration, intensity, and frequency of the physical activity in cancer protection needs to be further explored.

A number of different diets associated with cancer have been identified. Importantly, healthy fats (polysaturated and unsaturated fats), fruits, vegetables, and fibre does not appear to increase cancer risk[554].

Although the studies are not yet entirely conclusive, consuming different types of nutrients, micronutrients and various supplements appears to provide a certain protection against certain different types of cancers[555].

The positive effect of healthy fat is well-known factor in the geographic cancer rate differences globally. Although the data on prostate cancer are more convincing, the link between total fat intake and colon or breast cancer has not yet been found and established[556].

Although it has been debated[557], it has been suggested that a low fat diet controlled for caloric intake might be protective against colorectal cancer.

A low fat diet also tends to reduce breast cancer, especially for women who have a high fat intake prior to initiating the diet[558].

A high fat diet appears to be associated with the development of prostate cancer, especially consuming large amounts of alpha-linoleic acid and low amounts of linoleic acid, as in red meat and dairy products, appear to increase the risk[559]. This is probably partly due to the lower serum levels of testosterone that follow a decreased fat intake.

It is important to emphasise that observational and randomised controlled trials may result in inaccurate outcomes due to several factors, e.g. poor adherence to the specific diet at hand, inadequate follow-up time, incorrect dose of the specific diet, etc.

Also, most studies only focus on one specific type of diet with a single component, when a combination of several different nutrients in a healthy combination is probably better when assessing cancer risk.

However, one consistent finding is that excess calories from any source leads to weight gain and an increase in the risk of multiple types of cancers[560].

Fertility, pregnancy and obesity

Obesity during pregnancy is associated with countless risks to both mother and foetus. The increased level of obesity therefore increases the risk of developing problems such as diabetes[561-563]. Although it is challenging to the healthcare provider, managing the problems can significantly reduce their risk[564].

Although the prevalence of obesity is higher in reproductive and pregnant women, it varies considerably depending on a number of different characteristics and definitions[565-572].

Polycystic ovary syndrome is believed to be closely associated to obesity[573,574]. In women with regular ovulation, obesity is associated with decreased spontaneous pregnancies and increased time to pregnancy[575-577].

Prolonged, or post-term, pregnancy is closely associated with obesity[567,572,578,579], and obesity prior to pregnancy also significantly increases the need for caesarean delivery[580].

The risk of having to give birth through caesarean delivery increases with the level of obesity[581] and is independent of other obesity-related complications[571,582]. Gaining excessive weight prior to and during pregnancy also increases the risk of having to give birth through caesarean delivery[571,583,584].

Also, obese mothers stay significantly longer in the hospital after giving birth compared with non-obese mothers[585,586]. The reason for the longer hospitalisation is related to an increased number of postpartum complications, which in turn leads to increased health care costs[586,587].

Urology and obesity

The most commonly diagnosed urolological problems related to obesity are urinary incontinence and erectile dysfunction.

All types of incontinence are significantly more common in obese people[588]. Incontinence is twice as prevalent in obese compared to people with normal weight[589]. Therefore, weight loss greatly improves urinary incontinence[590].

As many as one third of obese men suffer from reversible erectile dysfunction, and losing weight will significantly improve sexual function[591]. Finally, the risk of renal failure increases three to four times in obese compared with normal weight people[592].

Mortality and obesity

Obesity is one of the leading preventable causes of death globally[593-595], and even though it is occasionally debated a large number of deaths are directly related to obesity[594,596].

Also, it is well recognised that high BMI inevitably results in shorter life expectancy[597-599]. Obesity reduces life expectancy by as many as six to seven years compared to healthy weight subjects[449,600]. Obesity and premature death are thus closely related and is thought to be as deadly, or even deadlier, than smoking[601].

The relationship between obesity and mortality is clearly established[602-613]. All-cause mortality is also reported to be higher in obese compared with normal weight people[614]. Higher BMI is thus associated with increased rate of death from all causes including cardiovascular disease.

The annual number of deaths attributable to obesity in the United States alone are thought to be as high as 365,000[615,616].

Non-smoking people who are 50 years old have an increased risk of death associated to overweight or obese, and with a BMI of ≥30 the risk increases more than threefold.

Also, the risk of all-cause mortality is independent of gender and ethnicity[604,617], and mortality is lowest among people with a BMI between 22.5 to 25, and the overall mortality increases with 30% when BMI increases to between 27.5 and 30[610]. Similarly, non-smoking patients who do not have heart disease or cancer have the lowest mortality risk.

For people with a BMI between 25 and 49.9 each increase of 5 BMI units, the mortality risk increases with 30%. This clearly confirms that being severely obese is seriously life-threatening[618]. In Asians the lowest risk of death is slightly decreased compared to people from other parts of the world, i.e. a BMI in the range of between 22.6 and 27.5[619].

Many different factors may partly explain the variability in the rates of overweight and obesity-related mortality, e.g. choice of statistical methods and different study populations[620].

A number of other factors that may influence mortality include age, gender, ethnicity, smoking, body fat distribution and other associated health conditions[621].

The term "metabolically healthy" obese and overweight is defined as individuals who do not have fat-associated cardiometabolic disorders, e.g. hypertension, hypertriglyceridaemia, low HDL cholesterol, impaired fasting glucose and insulin resistance[622].

Although obese people are at increased risk for developing long-term complications even in the absence of metabolic abnormalities, it has been debated if this also applies to metabolically healthy overweight individuals.

Metabolically healthy obese individuals have an increased mortality risk compared with those with normal weight[613]. However, it needs to be further investigated if this also applies to metabolically healthy overweight people. Also, most obese individuals become progressively less healthy over time[623].

Interestingly, people with BMI below 22.5 have higher mortality compared with subjects with a BMI of between 22.5 and 25, where the higher mortality in this group is, however, predominantly due to smoking-related disorders, e.g. cardiovascular, respiratory and cancer[610].

Asian people with BMI below 20.1 have considerably higher mortality than those with a BMI between 22.6 and 25, and in non-smoking Asians the risk is decreased [619].

Underweight is defined as a BMI <18.5, excluding subjects with illness-related weight loss[616]. Like being overweight and obese, being underweight is also associated with increased mortality in both smokers and non-smokers[616].

Although the association between BMI and cardiovascular disease mortality was weaker in South Asians, comparing a BMI of 22.5 with 24.9 in East Asians reveals a significantly increased risk of total cardiovascular death in those with higher BMI[624]. The same increased risk of cardiovascular mortality applies to East Asians with a BMI below 17.5.

Being overweight during adolescence, at age 18 years, increases the risk of premature death as an adult, and the risk further increases with a BMI greater than 25[369].

Trends in cardiovascular risk factors may appear a bit confusing since the prevalence of obesity (BMI >30) increased dramatically (from 15% – 30% in the United States from 1960 to 2000) while the mortality in obese people has decreased over time[616,625].

The reason for this is probably related to more aggressive and effective management of cardiovascular risk factors. These changes are seen in all weight groups, including obese individuals, and were associated with increases in the use of lipid-lowering drugs and antihypertensive medications.

During the same period, i.e. between 1960 and 2000, the increase in diagnosed type 2 diabetes increased from 1.8% to 5.0% and was most prominent in obese people, in which the increase was as high as from 2.9% to 10.1%[625].

As a result, the impact of obesity on mortality appeared to decrease over time[616]. However, the cardiovascular improvements have not been accompanied by reduced disability in obese people[626], suggesting that obese people are more likely than the non-obese to report various functional impairments throughout life.

However, other reports state that there is no evidence that the association between obesity and mortality have decreased over time[627].

The effect of fitness is an important factor in obese people. Compared to fit normal weight individuals, unfit individuals have twice the mortality risk regardless of their BMI[628]. Also, fit overweight and obese people have similar mortality risks compared with fit normal weight individuals.

Both obesity and low levels of physical activity are independent mortality predictors, so more physical activity alone may not influence the association between obesity and mortality[546,629].

Obesity in adulthood is also associated with a noticeable reduction in life expectancy. The lives of those who are severely obese may lose up to 8 years of their life, obese people can lose up to 6 years, and those who are overweight might lose up to three years[630].

Those who are both obese and smoke lose between 13 to 14 years of their lives compared with normal-weight non-smokers[600]. Obesity's influence on years of life lost is greater for men than for women and for white compared with black people[631].

Although smoking has been named the number one of the great causes of decreased life expectancy, the negative impact of obesity on life expectancy is predicted to surpass the health benefits of smoking cessation[599].

The steady rise in life expectancy during the past two centuries will probably come to an end and decrease because of the increasing prevalence of obesity[597].

ECONOMIC CONSEQUENCES

Economic consequences of obesity

Costs of obesity are logically classified as direct costs (medical and treatment-related costs), and indirect costs (other costs related to not being able to work etc.).

It is estimated that as much as 6 to 7% of total healthcare costs in developed countries is directly related to obesity[6].

In the US costs related to obesity amounts to 10% of the total healthcare costs[632]. However, the true costs, i.e. the combination between the direct and indirect costs, are of course considerably higher.

In 2008 in the US alone estimated annual costs of treating conditions directly related to obesity in adults was estimated to $147 billion[632]. The direct costs associated with obese outpatient children have been reported to be $14.1 billion[633].

However, the inpatient costs in childhood obesity amounts to as much as $200 to 237.6 billion[634,635].

This is not surprising since it has been reported that moderately obese people, i.e. with a BMI between 30 and 35, visit doctors 17% more, and severely obese people, i.e. with a BMI of 35 or higher, visit doctors 24% more compared with normal weight people[636]. Also, obese people use about 48% more inpatient days per year compared with normal weight people[637].

FINAL WORD

And a final word of wisdom….

Since the obesity pandemic has increased steadily since 1980, it is safe to assume that even if we find ways to limit or stop the increasing global obesity problem its consequences will continue to cause substantial health implications leading to unimaginable healthcare costs for a long time.

(… to be continued in volume 2. Prevention and treatment).

REFERENCES

1. American Medical Association. AMA adopts new policies on second day of voting at annual meeting [press release]. (June 18, 2013).
2. Must, A., *et al*. The disease burden associated with overweight and obesity. *JAMA* **282**, 1523-1529 (1999).
3. WHO. Fact sheet No. 311: Obesity and Overweight. (2013).
4. Åkesson, A., Larsson, S.C., Discacciati, A. & Wolk, A. Low-Risk Diet and Lifestyle Habits in the Primary Prevention of Myocardial Infarction in MenA Population-Based Prospective Cohort Study. *Journal of the American College of Cardiology* **64**, 1299-1306 (2014).
5. Hammond, R.A. & Levine, R. The economic impact of obesity in the United States. *Diabetes Metab Syndr Obes* **3**, 285-295 (2010).
6. WHO. Global strategy on diet, physical activity and health. (Geneva, 2003).
7. WHO. Obesity: Preventing and Managing the Global Epidemic. Report of a WHO Consultation. (Geneva, 2000).
8. Flier, J.S. Obesity wars: molecular progress confronts an expanding epidemic. *Cell* **116**, 337-350 (2004).
9. Guthrie, J.F., Lin, B.H. & Frazao, E. Role of food prepared away from home in the American diet, 1977-78 versus 1994-96: changes and consequences. *Journal of nutrition education and behavior* **34**, 140-150 (2002).
10. Ogden, C.L., Flegal, K.M., Carroll, M.D. & Johnson, C.L. Prevalence and trends in overweight among US children and adolescents, 1999-2000. *JAMA* **288**, 1728-1732 (2002).
11. Strauss, R.S. & Pollack, H.A. Epidemic increase in childhood overweight, 1986-1998. *JAMA* **286**, 2845-2848 (2001).
12. Jolliffe, D. Extent of overweight among US children and adolescents from 1971 to 2000. *International journal of obesity and related metabolic disorders : journal of the International Association for the Study of Obesity* **28**, 4-9 (2004).
13. Dietz, W.H. & Robinson, T.N. Clinical practice. Overweight children and adolescents. *N Engl J Med* **352**, 2100-2109 (2005).
14. National Institutes of Health. Clinical Guidelines on the Identification, Evaluation, and Treatment of Overweight and Obesity in Adults--The Evidence Report. *Obes Res* **6** Suppl 2, 51S-209S (1998).
15. Deurenberg, P., Weststrate, J.A. & Seidell, J.C. Body mass index as a measure of body fatness: age- and sex-specific prediction formulas. *The British journal of nutrition* **65**, 105-114 (1991).
16. Flodmark, C.E., Lissau, I., Moreno, L.A., Pietrobelli, A. & Widhalm, K. New insights into the field of children and adolescents' obesity: the European

perspective. *International journal of obesity and related metabolic disorders : journal of the International Association for the Study of Obesity* **28**, 1189-1196 (2004).

17. Ashwell, M., Gunn, P. & Gibson, S. Waist-to-height ratio is a better screening tool than waist circumference and BMI for adult cardiometabolic risk factors: systematic review and meta-analysis. *Obesity reviews : an official journal of the International Association for the Study of Obesity* **13**, 275-286 (2012).

18. WHO. Preventing Chronic Diseases: a vital investment. (Geneva, 2005).

19. Baker, S., Overweight children and adolescents: a clinical report of the North American Society for Pediatric Gastroenterology, Hepatology and Nutrition. *Journal of pediatric gastroenterology and nutrition* **40**, 533-543 (2005).

20. WHO. BMI-for-age (5-19 years). (Geneva, 2007).

21. WHO. World Health Statistics. (Geneva, 2009).

22. WHO. BMI Classification. Global Database on Body Mass Index. (World Health Organisation, Updated 26 may, 2014).

23. Yu, Z., *et al.* Pre-pregnancy body mass index in relation to infant birth weight and offspring overweight/obesity: a systematic review and meta-analysis. *PLoS One* **8**, e61627 (2013).

24. Power, C. & Jefferis, B.J. Fetal environment and subsequent obesity: a study of maternal smoking. *International journal of epidemiology* **31**, 413-419 (2002).

25. Dabelea, D., *et al.* Intrauterine exposure to diabetes conveys risks for type 2 diabetes and obesity: a study of discordant sibships. *Diabetes* **49**, 2208-2211 (2000).

26. Toschke, A.M., Ehlin, A.G., von Kries, R., Ekbom, A. & Montgomery, S.M. Maternal smoking during pregnancy and appetite control in offspring. *Journal of perinatal medicine* **31**, 251-256 (2003).

27. de Boo, H.A. & Harding, J.E. The developmental origins of adult disease (Barker) hypothesis. *The Australian & New Zealand journal of obstetrics & gynaecology* **46**, 4-14 (2006).

28. Wilson, R.S. Concordance in physical growth for monozygotic and dizygotic twins. *Ann Hum Biol* **3**, 1-10 (1976).

29. Bray, G.A. & Bellanger, T. Epidemiology, trends, and morbidities of obesity and the metabolic syndrome. *Endocrine* **29**, 109-117 (2006).

30. Hediger, M.L., Overpeck, M.D., Kuczmarski, R.J. & Ruan, W.J. Association between infant breastfeeding and overweight in young children. *JAMA* **285**, 2453-2460 (2001).

31. Gillman, M.W., *et al.* Risk of overweight among adolescents who were breastfed as infants. *JAMA* **285**, 2461-2467 (2001).

32. von Kries, R., *et al.* Breast feeding and obesity: cross sectional study. *BMJ* **319**, 147-150 (1999).

33. Harder, T., Bergmann, R., Kallischnigg, G. & Plagemann, A. Duration of breastfeeding and risk of overweight: a meta-analysis. *Am J Epidemiol* **162**, 397-403 (2005).

34. Whitaker, R.C., Wright, J.A., Pepe, M.S., Seidel, K.D. & Dietz, W.H. Predicting obesity in young adulthood from childhood and parental obesity. *N Engl J Med* **337**, 869-873 (1997).

35. The, N.S., Suchindran, C., North, K.E., Popkin, B.M. & Gordon-Larsen, P. Association of adolescent obesity with risk of severe obesity in adulthood. *JAMA* **304**, 2042-2047 (2010).

36. Must, A., Phillips, S.M. & Naumova, E.N. Occurrence and timing of childhood overweight and mortality: findings from the Third Harvard Growth Study. *J Pediatr* **160**, 743-750 (2012).

37. Bray, G.A. The obese patient. in *Major problems in internal medicine* (WB Saunders, , Philadelphia, 1976).

38. Freedman, D.S., Mei, Z., Srinivasan, S.R., Berenson, G.S. & Dietz, W.H. Cardiovascular risk factors and excess adiposity among overweight children and adolescents: the Bogalusa Heart Study. *J Pediatr* **150**, 12-17 e12 (2007).

39. Skelton, J.A., Cook, S.R., Auinger, P., Klein, J.D. & Barlow, S.E. Prevalence and trends of severe obesity among US children and adolescents. *Academic pediatrics* **9**, 322-329 (2009).

40. Barlow, S.E. & Expert, C. Expert committee recommendations regarding the prevention, assessment, and treatment of child and adolescent overweight and obesity: summary report. *Pediatrics* **120 Suppl** 4, S164-192 (2007).

41. Prentice, A.M. & Jebb, S.A. Obesity in Britain: gluttony or sloth? *BMJ* **311**, 437-439 (1995).

42. Kromhout, D. Changes in energy and macronutrients in 871 middle-aged men during 10 years of follow-up (the Zutphen study). *Am J Clin Nutr* **37**, 287-294 (1983).

43. Williamson, D.F., *et al.* Recreational physical activity and ten-year weight change in a US national cohort. *International journal of obesity and related metabolic disorders : journal of the International Association for the Study of Obesity* **17**, 279-286 (1993).

44. Hu, F.B., Li, T.Y., Colditz, G.A., Willett, W.C. & Manson, J.E. Television watching and other sedentary behaviors in relation to risk of obesity and type 2 diabetes mellitus in women. *JAMA* **289**, 1785-1791 (2003).

45. Dietz, W.H., Jr. & Gortmaker, S.L. Do we fatten our children at the television set? Obesity and television viewing in children and adolescents. *Pediatrics* **75**, 807-812 (1985).

46. Gortmaker, S.L., *et al.* Television viewing as a cause of increasing obesity among children in the United States, 1986-1990. *Arch Pediatr Adolesc Med* **150**, 356-362 (1996).

47. Kaur, H., Choi, W.S., Mayo, M.S. & Harris, K.J. Duration of television watching is associated with increased body mass index. *J Pediatr* **143**, 506-511 (2003).

48. Berkey, C.S., Rockett, H.R., Gillman, M.W. & Colditz, G.A. One-year changes in activity and in inactivity among 10- to 15-year-old boys and girls: relationship to change in body mass index. *Pediatrics* **111**, 836-843 (2003).

49. Blair, N.J., *et al.* Risk factors for obesity in 7-year-old European children: the Auckland Birthweight Collaborative Study. *Arch Dis Child* **92**, 866-871 (2007).

50. Hancox, R.J., Milne, B.J. & Poulton, R. Association between child and adolescent

television viewing and adult health: a longitudinal birth cohort study. *Lancet* **364**, 257-262 (2004).

51. Viner, R.M. & Cole, T.J. Television viewing in early childhood predicts adult body mass index. *J Pediatr* **147**, 429-435 (2005).

52. Marshall, S.J., Biddle, S.J., Gorely, T., Cameron, N. & Murdey, I. Relationships between media use, body fatness and physical activity in children and youth: a meta-analysis. *International journal of obesity and related metabolic disorders : journal of the International Association for the Study of Obesity* **28**, 1238-1246 (2004).

53. Wake, M., Hesketh, K. & Waters, E. Television, computer use and body mass index in Australian primary school children. *Journal of paediatrics and child health* **39**, 130-134 (2003).

54. Wahi, G., Parkin, P.C., Beyene, J., Uleryk, E.M. & Birken, C.S. Effectiveness of interventions aimed at reducing screen time in children: a systematic review and meta-analysis of randomized controlled trials. *Arch Pediatr Adolesc Med* **165**, 979-986 (2011).

55. Ludwig, D.S. & Gortmaker, S.L. Programming obesity in childhood. *Lancet* **364**, 226-227 (2004).

56. Boyland, E.J., *et al.* Food commercials increase preference for energy-dense foods, particularly in children who watch more television. Pediatrics 128, e93-100 (2011).

57. Epstein, L.H., *et al.* A randomized trial of the effects of reducing television viewing and computer use on body mass index in young children. *Arch Pediatr Adolesc Med* **162**, 239-245 (2008).

58. Lipsky, L.M. & Iannotti, R.J. Associations of television viewing with eating behaviors in the 2009 Health Behaviour in School-aged Children Study. *Arch Pediatr Adolesc Med* **166**, 465-472 (2012).

59. Epstein, L.H., Roemmich, J.N., Paluch, R.A. & Raynor, H.A. Influence of changes in sedentary behavior on energy and macronutrient intake in youth. *Am J Clin Nutr* **81**, 361-366 (2005).

60. Stettler, N., Signer, T.M. & Suter, P.M. Electronic games and environmental factors associated with childhood obesity in Switzerland. *Obes Res* **12**, 896-903 (2004).

61. Kautiainen, S., Koivusilta, L., Lintonen, T., Virtanen, S.M. & Rimpela, A. Use of information and communication technology and prevalence of overweight and obesity among adolescents. *International journal of obesity* **29**, 925-933 (2005).

62. Bickham, D.S., Blood, E.A., Walls, C.E., Shrier, L.A. & Rich, M. Characteristics of screen media use associated with higher BMI in young adolescents. *Pediatrics* **131**, 935-941 (2013).

63. Brown, D. Playing to win: video games and the fight against obesity. *Journal of the American Dietetic Association* **106**, 188-189 (2006).

64. Baranowski, T., *et al.* Squire's Quest! Dietary outcome evaluation of a multimedia game. *Am J Prev Med* **24**, 52-61 (2003).

65. Lanningham-Foster, L., *et al.* Energy expenditure of sedentary screen time compared with active screen time for children. *Pediatrics* **118**, e1831-1835 (2006).

66. Mellecker, R.R. & McManus, A.M. Energy expenditure and cardiovascular responses to seated and active gaming in children. *Arch Pediatr Adolesc Med* **162**, 886-891 (2008).

67. Graf, D.L., Pratt, L.V., Hester, C.N. & Short, K.R. Playing active video games increases energy expenditure in children. *Pediatrics* **124**, 534-540 (2009).

68. Biddiss, E. & Irwin, J. Active video games to promote physical activity in children

and youth: a systematic review. *Arch Pediatr Adolesc Med* **164**, 664-672 (2010).

69. O'Loughlin, E.K., Dugas, E.N., Sabiston, C.M. & O'Loughlin, J.L. Prevalence and correlates of exergaming in youth. *Pediatrics* **130**, 806-814 (2012).

70. Graves, L., Stratton, G., Ridgers, N.D. & Cable, N.T. Comparison of energy expenditure in adolescents when playing new generation and sedentary computer games: cross sectional study. *BMJ* **335**, 1282-1284 (2007).

71. Bailey, B.W. & McInnis, K. Energy cost of exergaming: a comparison of the energy cost of 6 forms of exergaming. *Arch Pediatr Adolesc Med* **165**, 597-602 (2011).

72. Madsen, K.A., Yen, S., Wlasiuk, L., Newman, T.B. & Lustig, R. Feasibility of a dance videogame to promote weight loss among overweight children and adolescents. *Arch Pediatr Adolesc Med* **161**, 105-107 (2007).

73. Christison, A. & Khan, H.A. Exergaming for health: a community-based pediatric weight management program using active video gaming. *Clin Pediatr (Phila)* **51**, 382-388 (2012).

74. Weil, E., *et al.* Obesity among adults with disabling conditions. *JAMA* **288**, 1265-1268 (2002).

75. Anderson, S.E. & Whitaker, R.C. Household routines and obesity in US preschool-aged children. *Pediatrics* **125**, 420-428 (2010).

76. Chaput, J.P. & Tremblay, A. Does short sleep duration favor abdominal adiposity in children? *International journal of pediatric obesity : IJPO : an official journal of the International Association for the Study of Obesity* **2**, 188-191 (2007).

77. Flint, J., *et al.* Association between inadequate sleep and insulin resistance in obese children. *J Pediatr* **150**, 364-369 (2007).

78. Sekine, M., *et al.* A dose-response relationship between short sleeping hours and childhood obesity: results of the Toyama Birth Cohort Study. *Child: care, health and development* **28**, 163-170 (2002).

79. Jiang, F., *et al.* Sleep and obesity in preschool children. *J Pediatr* **154**, 814-818 (2009).

80. Altenburg, T.M., *et al.* Longer sleep--slimmer kids: the ENERGY-project. *PLoS One* **8**, e59522 (2013).

81. Bayer, O., Rosario, A.S., Wabitsch, M. & von Kries, R. Sleep duration and obesity in children: is the association dependent on age and choice of the outcome parameter? *Sleep* **32**, 1183-1189 (2009).

82. Cappuccio, F.P., *et al.* Meta-analysis of short sleep duration and obesity in children and adults. *Sleep* **31**, 619-626 (2008).

83. Lumeng, J.C., *et al.* Shorter sleep duration is associated with increased risk for being overweight at ages 9 to 12 years. Pediatrics 120, 1020-1029 (2007).

84. Landhuis, C.E., Poulton, R., Welch, D. & Hancox, R.J. Childhood sleep time and long-term risk for obesity: a 32-year prospective birth cohort study. *Pediatrics* **122**, 955-960 (2008).

85. Touchette, E., *et al.* Associations between sleep duration patterns and overweight/ obesity at age 6. *Sleep* **31**, 1507-1514 (2008).

86. Carter, P.J., Taylor, B.J., Williams, S.M. & Taylor, R.W. Longitudinal analysis of sleep in relation to BMI and body fat in children: the FLAME study. *BMJ* **342**, d2712 (2011).

87. Araujo, J., Severo, M. & Ramos, E. Sleep duration and adiposity during adolescence. *Pediatrics* **130**, e1146-1154 (2012).

88. Hiscock, H., Scalzo, K., Canterford, L. & Wake, M. Sleep duration and body mass

index in 0-7-year olds. *Arch Dis Child* **96**, 735-739 (2011).

89. Lesser, D.J., *et al.* Sleep fragmentation and intermittent hypoxemia are associated with decreased insulin sensitivity in obese adolescent Latino males. *Pediatr Res* **72**, 293-298 (2012).

90. Koren, D., *et al.* Sleep architecture and glucose and insulin homeostasis in obese adolescents. *Diabetes Care* **34**, 2442-2447 (2011).

91. Filozof, C., Fernandez Pinilla, M.C. & Fernandez-Cruz, A. Smoking cessation and weight gain. *Obesity reviews : an official journal of the International Association for the Study of Obesity* **5**, 95-103 (2004).

92. Leslie, W.S., *et al.* Changes in body weight and food choice in those attempting smoking cessation: a cluster randomised controlled trial. *BMC public health* **12**, 389 (2012).

93. Eisen, S.A., Lyons, M.J., Goldberg, J. & True, W.R. The impact of cigarette and alcohol consumption on weight and obesity. An analysis of 1911 monozygotic male twin pairs. *Arch Intern Med* **153**, 2457-2463 (1993).

94. Parsons, T.J., Power, C., Logan, S. & Summerbell, C.D. Childhood predictors of adult obesity: a systematic review. *International journal of obesity and related metabolic disorders : journal of the International Association for the Study of Obesity* **23 Suppl 8**, S1-107 (1999).

95. Plachta-Danielzik, S., *et al.* Attributable risks for childhood overweight: evidence for limited effectiveness of prevention. *Pediatrics* **130**, e865-871 (2012).

96. Taber, D.R., Chriqui, J.F., Powell, L. & Chaloupka, F.J. Association between state laws governing school meal nutrition content and student weight status: implications for new USDA school meal standards. *JAMA pediatrics* **167**, 513-519 (2013).

97. Bremer, A.A., Auinger, P. & Byrd, R.S. Relationship between insulin resistance-associated metabolic parameters and anthropometric measurements with sugar-sweetened beverage intake and physical activity levels in US adolescents: findings from the 1999-2004 National Health and Nutrition Examination Survey. *Arch Pediatr Adolesc Med* **163**, 328-335 (2009).

98. Malik, V.S., Schulze, M.B. & Hu, F.B. Intake of sugar-sweetened beverages and weight gain: a systematic review. *Am J Clin Nutr* **84**, 274-288 (2006).

99. Berkey, C.S., Rockett, H.R., Field, A.E., Gillman, M.W. & Colditz, G.A. Sugar-added beverages and adolescent weight change. *Obes Res* **12**, 778-788 (2004).

100. Ebbeling, C.B., *et al.* Effects of decreasing sugar-sweetened beverage consumption on body weight in adolescents: a randomized, controlled pilot study. *Pediatrics* **117**, 673-680 (2006).

101. Dowda, M., Ainsworth, B.E., Addy, C.L., Saunders, R. & Riner, W. Environmental influences, physical activity, and weight status in 8- to 16-year-olds. *Arch Pediatr Adolesc Med* **155**, 711-717 (2001).

102. Menschik, D., Ahmed, S., Alexander, M.H. & Blum, R.W. Adolescent physical activities as predictors of young adult weight. *Arch Pediatr Adolesc Med* **162**, 29-33 (2008).

103. Levin, S., Lowry, R., Brown, D.R. & Dietz, W.H. Physical activity and body mass index among US adolescents: youth risk behavior survey, 1999. *Arch Pediatr Adolesc Med* **157**, 816-820 (2003).

104. Drake, K.M., *et al.* Influence of sports, physical education, and active commuting to school on adolescent weight status. *Pediatrics* **130**, e296-304 (2012).

105. Dhingra, R., *et al.* Soft drink consumption and risk of developing cardiometabolic risk factors and the metabolic syndrome in middle-aged adults in the community. *Circulation* **116**, 480-488 (2007).

106. Tetri, L.H., Basaranoglu, M., Brunt, E.M., Yerian, L.M. & Neuschwander-Tetri, B.A. Severe NAFLD with hepatic necroinflammatory changes in mice fed trans fats and a high-fructose corn syrup equivalent. *American journal of physiology. Gastrointestinal and liver physiology* **295**, G987-995 (2008).

107. Basaranoglu, M., Basaranoglu, G., Sabuncu, T. & Senturk, H. Fructose as a key player in the development of fatty liver disease. *World journal of gastroenterology : WJG* **19**, 1166-1172 (2013).

108. Waters, E., *et al.* Interventions for preventing obesity in children. Cochrane Database Syst Rev, CD001871 (2011).

109. Konttinen, H., Haukkala, A., Sarlio-Lahteenkorva, S., Silventoinen, K. & Jousilahti, P. Eating styles, self-control and obesity indicators. The moderating role of obesity status and dieting history on restrained eating. *Appetite* **53**, 131-134 (2009).

110. Bouchard, C., *et al.* The response to long-term overfeeding in identical twins. *N Engl J Med* **322**, 1477-1482 (1990).

111. Lawson, O.J., *et al.* The association of body weight, dietary intake, and energy expenditure with dietary restraint and disinhibition. *Obes Res* **3**, 153-161 (1995).

112. Jaaskelainen, A., *et al.* Associations of meal frequency and breakfast with obesity and metabolic syndrome traits in adolescents of Northern Finland Birth Cohort 1986. *Nutrition, metabolism, and cardiovascular diseases : NMCD* (2012).

113. Toschke, A.M., Thorsteinsdottir, K.H., von Kries, R. & Group, G.M.E.S. Meal frequency, breakfast consumption and childhood obesity. *International journal of pediatric obesity : IJPO : an official journal of the International Association for the Study of Obesity* **4**, 242-248 (2009).

114. Rampersaud, G.C., Pereira, M.A., Girard, B.L., Adams, J. & Metzl, J.D. Breakfast habits, nutritional status, body weight, and academic performance in children and adolescents. *Journal of the American Dietetic Association* **105**, 743-760; quiz 761-742 (2005).

115. Jenkins, D.J., *et al.* Nibbling versus gorging: metabolic advantages of increased meal frequency. *N Engl J Med* **321**, 929-934 (1989).

116. Bray, G.A. & Popkin, B.M. Dietary fat intake does affect obesity! *Am J Clin Nutr* **68**, 1157-1173 (1998).

117. Mozaffarian, D., Hao, T., Rimm, E.B., Willett, W.C. & Hu, F.B. Changes in diet and lifestyle and long-term weight gain in women and men. *N Engl J Med* **364**, 2392-2404 (2011).

118. Qi, Q., *et al.* Sugar-sweetened beverages and genetic risk of obesity. *N Engl J Med* **367**, 1387-1396 (2012).

119. McCaffery, J.M., *et al.* Obesity susceptibility loci and dietary intake in the Look AHEAD Trial. *Am J Clin Nutr* **95**, 1477-1486 (2012).

120. Wang, Y.C., Bleich, S.N. & Gortmaker, S.L. Increasing caloric contribution from sugar-sweetened beverages and 100% fruit juices among US children and adolescents, 1988-2004. *Pediatrics* **121**, e1604-1614 (2008).

121. Ebbeling, C.B., *et al.* A randomized trial of sugar-sweetened beverages and adolescent body weight. *N Engl J Med* **367**, 1407-1416 (2012).

122. de Ruyter, J.C., Olthof, M.R., Seidell, J.C. & Katan, M.B. A trial of sugar-free or

sugar-sweetened beverages and body weight in children. *N Engl J Med* **367**, 1397-1406 (2012).

123. Farley, T.A. The role of government in preventing excess calorie consumption: the example of New York City. *JAMA* **308**, 1093-1094 (2012).

124. Elbel, B., Cantor, J. & Mijanovich, T. Potential effect of the New York City policy regarding sugared beverages. *N Engl J Med* **367**, 680-681 (2012).

125. Turner, L. & Chaloupka, F.J. Encouraging trends in student access to competitive beverages in US public elementary schools, 2006-2007 to 2010-2011. *Arch Pediatr Adolesc Med* **166**, 673-675 (2012).

126. Pomeranz, J.L. & Brownell, K.D. Portion sizes and beyond--government's legal authority to regulate food-industry practices. *N Engl J Med* **367**, 1383-1385 (2012).

127. Grimes, C.A., Riddell, L.J., Campbell, K.J. & Nowson, C.A. Dietary salt intake, sugar-sweetened beverage consumption, and obesity risk. *Pediatrics* **131**, 14-21 (2013).

128. Grimes, C.A., Wright, J.D., Liu, K., Nowson, C.A. & Loria, C.M. Dietary sodium intake is associated with total fluid and sugar-sweetened beverage consumption in US children and adolescents aged 2-18 y: NHANES 2005-2008. *Am J Clin Nutr* **98**, 189-196 (2013).

129. Fernstrom, M.H. Drugs that cause weight gain. *Obes Res* **3** Suppl 4, 435S-439S (1995).

130. Leslie, W.S., Hankey, C.R. & Lean, M.E. Weight gain as an adverse effect of some commonly prescribed drugs: a systematic review. *QJM : monthly journal of the Association of Physicians* **100**, 395-404 (2007).

131. Fava, M. Weight gain and antidepressants. *J Clin Psychiatry* **61 Suppl 11**, 37-41 (2000).

132. Fava, M., Judge, R., Hoog, S.L., Nilsson, M.E. & Koke, S.C. Fluoxetine versus sertraline and paroxetine in major depressive disorder: changes in weight with long-term treatment. *J Clin Psychiatry* **61**, 863-867 (2000).

133. Ogden, C.L., Carroll, M.D., Kit, B.K. & Flegal, K.M. Prevalence of obesity and trends in body mass index among US children and adolescents, 1999-2010. *JAMA* **307**, 483-490 (2012).

134. Kelly, A.S., *et al.* Severe Obesity in Children and Adolescents: Identification, Associated Health Risks, and Treatment Approaches: A Scientific Statement From the American Heart Association. *Circulation* (2013).

135. Claire Wang, Y., Gortmaker, S.L. & Taveras, E.M. Trends and racial/ethnic disparities in severe obesity among US children and adolescents, 1976-2006. *International journal of pediatric obesity : IJPO : an official journal of the International Association for the Study of Obesity* **6**, 12-20 (2011).

136. Anderson, S.E. & Whitaker, R.C. Prevalence of obesity among US preschool children in different racial and ethnic groups. *Arch Pediatr Adolesc Med* **163**, 344-348 (2009).

137. Taveras, E.M., Gillman, M.W., Kleinman, K., Rich-Edwards, J.W. & Rifas-Shiman, S.L. Racial/ethnic differences in early-life risk factors for childhood obesity. *Pediatrics* **125**, 686-695 (2010).

138. Pan, L., Blanck, H.M., Sherry, B., Dalenius, K. & Grummer-Strawn, L.M. Trends in the prevalence of extreme obesity among US preschool-aged children living in low-income families, 1998-2010. *JAMA* **308**, 2563-2565 (2012).

139. Eagle, T.F., *et al.* Understanding childhood obesity in America: linkages between household income, community resources, and children's behaviors. *Am Heart J* **163**, 836-843 (2012).

140. Neovius, M., Linne, Y., Barkeling, B. & Rossner, S. Discrepancies between classification systems of childhood obesity. *Obesity reviews : an official journal of the International Association for the Study of Obesity* **5**, 105-114 (2004).

141. Wang, Y. Cross-national comparison of childhood obesity: the epidemic and the relationship between obesity and socioeconomic status. *International journal of epidemiology* **30**, 1129-1136 (2001).

142. Janssen, I., *et al.* Comparison of overweight and obesity prevalence in school-aged youth from 34 countries and their relationships with physical activity and dietary patterns. *Obesity reviews : an official journal of the International Association for the Study of Obesity* **6**, 123-132 (2005).

143. Wang, G. & Dietz, W.H. Economic burden of obesity in youths aged 6 to 17 years: 1979-1999. *Pediatrics* **109**, E81-81 (2002).

144. Madsen, K.A., Weedn, A.E. & Crawford, P.B. Disparities in peaks, plateaus, and declines in prevalence of high BMI among adolescents. *Pediatrics* **126**, 434-442 (2010).

145. Aeberli, I., Ammann, R.S., Knabenhans, M., Molinari, L. & Zimmermann, M.B. Decrease in the prevalence of paediatric adiposity in Switzerland from 2002 to 2007. *Public Health Nutr* **13**, 806-811 (2010).

146. Wen, X., *et al.* Decreasing prevalence of obesity among young children in Massachusetts from 2004 to 2008. *Pediatrics* **129**, 823-831 (2012).

147. Olds, T.S., Tomkinson, G.R., Ferrar, K.E. & Maher, C.A. Trends in the prevalence of childhood overweight and obesity in Australia between 1985 and 2008. *International journal of obesity* **34**, 57-66 (2010).

148. Salanave, B., Peneau, S., Rolland-Cachera, M.F., Hercberg, S. & Castetbon, K. Stabilization of overweight prevalence in French children between 2000 and 2007. *International journal of pediatric obesity : IJPO : an official journal of the International Association for the Study of Obesity* **4**, 66-72 (2009).

149. Guo, S.S., Roche, A.F., Chumlea, W.C., Gardner, J.D. & Siervogel, R.M. The predictive value of childhood body mass index values for overweight at age 35 y. *Am J Clin Nutr* **59**, 810-819 (1994).

150. Power, C., Lake, J.K. & Cole, T.J. Body mass index and height from childhood to adulthood in the 1958 British born cohort. *Am J Clin Nutr* **66**, 1094-1101 (1997).

151. Parsons, A.C., Shraim, M., Inglis, J., Aveyard, P. & Hajek, P. Interventions for preventing weight gain after smoking cessation. *Cochrane Database Syst Rev*, CD006219 (2009).

152. Reilly, J.J., *et al.* Health consequences of obesity. *Arch Dis Child* **88**, 748-752 (2003).

153. Whitlock, E.P., Williams, S.B., Gold, R., Smith, P. & Shipman, S. *Screening and Interventions for Childhood Overweight*, (Rockville (MD), 2005).

154. Garn, S.M. & LaVelle, M. Two-decade follow-up of fatness in early childhood. *Am J Dis Child* **139**, 181-185 (1985).

155. Juonala, M., *et al.* Childhood adiposity, adult adiposity, and cardiovascular risk factors. *N Engl J Med* **365**, 1876-1885 (2011).

156. Gulati, A.K., Kaplan, D.W. & Daniels, S.R. Clinical tracking of severely obese children: a new growth chart. *Pediatrics* **130**, 1136-1140 (2012).

157. Garn, S.M. & Cole, P.E. Do the obese remain obese and the lean remain lean? *American journal of public health* **70**, 351-353 (1980).
158. Mellits, E.D. & Cheek, D.B. The assessment of body water and fatness from infancy to adulthood. *Monographs of the Society for Research in Child Development* **35**, 12-26 (1970).
159. Deshmukh-Taskar, P., *et al.* Tracking of overweight status from childhood to young adulthood: the Bogalusa Heart Study. *Eur J Clin Nutr* **60**, 48-57 (2006).
160. Herman, K.M., Craig, C.L., Gauvin, L. & Katzmarzyk, P.T. Tracking of obesity and physical activity from childhood to adulthood: the Physical Activity Longitudinal Study. *International journal of pediatric obesity : IJPO : an official journal of the International Association for the Study of Obesity* **4**, 281-288 (2009).
161. Patton, G.C., *et al.* Overweight and obesity between adolescence and young adulthood: a 10-year prospective cohort study. *The Journal of adolescent health : official publication of the Society for Adolescent Medicine* **48**, 275-280 (2011).
162. Drewnowski, A., Rehm, C.D. & Solet, D. Disparities in obesity rates: analysis by ZIP code area. *Social science & medicine* **65**, 2458-2463 (2007).
163. Drewnowski, A. The economics of food choice behavior: why poverty and obesity are linked. *Nestle Nutrition Institute workshop series* **73**, 95-112 (2012).
164. Dubowitz, T., Ghosh-Dastidar, M.B., Steiner, E., Escarce, J.J. & Collins, R.L. Are our actions aligned with our evidence? The skinny on changing the landscape of obesity. *Obesity* **21**, 419-420 (2013).
165. McTigue, K.M., Garrett, J.M. & Popkin, B.M. The natural history of the development of obesity in a cohort of young U.S. adults between 1981 and 1998. *Ann Intern Med* **136**, 857-864 (2002).
166. Guyenet, S.J. & Schwartz, M.W. Clinical review: Regulation of food intake, energy balance, and body fat mass: implications for the pathogenesis and treatment of obesity. *J Clin Endocrinol Metab* **97**, 745-755 (2012).
167. Yu, J.H. & Kim, M.S. Molecular mechanisms of appetite regulation. *Diabetes & metabolism journal* **36**, 391-398 (2012).
168. Day, F.R. & Loos, R.J. Developments in obesity genetics in the era of genome-wide association studies. *Journal of nutrigenetics and nutrigenomics* **4**, 222-238 (2011).
169. Shang, Q., *et al.* Serological data analyses show that adenovirus 36 infection is associated with obesity: a meta-analysis involving 5739 subjects. *Obesity* **22**, 895-900 (2014).
170. de Ferranti, S. & Mozaffarian, D. The perfect storm: obesity, adipocyte dysfunction, and metabolic consequences. *Clin Chem* **54**, 945-955 (2008).
171. Bowman, S.A. & Vinyard, B.T. Fast food consumption of U.S. adults: impact on energy and nutrient intakes and overweight status. *J Am Coll Nutr* **23**, 163-168 (2004).
172. Paeratakul, S., Ferdinand, D.P., Champagne, C.M., Ryan, D.H. & Bray, G.A. Fast-food consumption among US adults and children: dietary and nutrient intake profile. *Journal of the American Dietetic Association* **103**, 1332-1338 (2003).
173. Britton, K.A., *et al.* Body fat distribution, incident cardiovascular disease, cancer, and all-cause mortality. *J Am Coll Cardiol* **62**, 921-925 (2013).
174. Oken, E., Taveras, E.M., Kleinman, K.P., Rich-Edwards, J.W. & Gillman, M.W. Gestational weight gain and child adiposity at age 3 years. *Am J Obstet Gynecol* **196**, 322 e321-328 (2007).

175. Baptiste-Roberts, K., Nicholson, W.K., Wang, N.Y. & Brancati, F.L. Gestational diabetes and subsequent growth patterns of offspring: the National Collaborative Perinatal Project. *Maternal and child health journal* **16**, 125-132 (2012).

176. Bray, G.A. *A Guide to Obesity and the Metabolic Syndrome*, (CRC Press, Boca Raton, FL., 2011).

177. Oken, E., Levitan, E.B. & Gillman, M.W. Maternal smoking during pregnancy and child overweight: systematic review and meta-analysis. *International journal of obesity* **32**, 201-210 (2008).

178. Loos, R.J. Genetic determinants of common obesity and their value in prediction. *Best practice & research. Clinical endocrinology & metabolism* **26**, 211-226 (2012).

179. Mannan, M., Doi, S.A. & Mamun, A.A. Association between weight gain during pregnancy and postpartum weight retention and obesity: a bias-adjusted meta-analysis. *Nutrition reviews* **71**, 343-352 (2013).

180. Smith, D.E., *et al.* Longitudinal changes in adiposity associated with pregnancy. The CARDIA Study. Coronary Artery Risk Development in Young Adults Study. *JAMA* **271**, 1747-1751 (1994).

181. Gunderson, E.P., *et al.* Childbearing may increase visceral adipose tissue independent of overall increase in body fat. *Obesity* **16**, 1078-1084 (2008).

182. Robinson, W.R., Cheng, M.M., Hoggatt, K.J., Sturmer, T. & Siega-Riz, A.M. Childbearing is not associated with young women's long-term obesity risk. *Obesity* **22**, 1126-1132 (2014).

183. Lovejoy, J.C. The menopause and obesity. *Primary care* **30**, 317-325 (2003).

184. Sowers, M., *et al.* Changes in body composition in women over six years at midlife: ovarian and chronological aging. *J Clin Endocrinol Metab* **92**, 895-901 (2007).

185. Berthoud, H.R. & Morrison, C. The brain, appetite, and obesity. *Annual review of psychology* **59**, 55-92 (2008).

186. Leibel, R.L., Rosenbaum, M. & Hirsch, J. Changes in energy expenditure resulting from altered body weight. *N Engl J Med* **332**, 621-628 (1995).

187. Van Wymelbeke, V., Brondel, L., Marcel Brun, J. & Rigaud, D. Factors associated with the increase in resting energy expenditure during refeeding in malnourished anorexia nervosa patients. *Am J Clin Nutr* **80**, 1469-1477 (2004).

188. Heymsfield, S.B., *et al.* Why do obese patients not lose more weight when treated with low-calorie diets? A mechanistic perspective. *Am J Clin Nutr* **85**, 346-354 (2007).

189. Gropper, S.S. & Smith, J.L. *Advanced Nutrition and Human Metabolism*, (Cengage Learning, 2012).

190. Gesta, S., Tseng, Y.H. & Kahn, C.R. Developmental origin of fat: tracking obesity to its source. *Cell* **131**, 242-256 (2007).

191. Cannon, B. & Nedergaard, J. Brown adipose tissue: function and physiological significance. *Physiol Rev* **84**, 277-359 (2004).

192. Drubach, L.A., *et al.* Pediatric brown adipose tissue: detection, epidemiology, and differences from adults. *J Pediatr* **159**, 939-944 (2011).

193. van Marken Lichtenbelt, W.D., *et al.* Cold-activated brown adipose tissue in healthy men. *N Engl J Med* **360**, 1500-1508 (2009).

194. Cypess, A.M., *et al.* Identification and importance of brown adipose tissue in adult humans. *N Engl J Med* **360**, 1509-1517 (2009).

195. Virtanen, K.A., *et al.* Functional brown adipose tissue in healthy adults. *N Engl J*

Med **360**, 1518-1525 (2009).

196. Ouellet, V., *et al.* Brown adipose tissue oxidative metabolism contributes to energy expenditure during acute cold exposure in humans. *The Journal of clinical investigation* **122**, 545-552 (2012).

197. Jensen, M.D. Role of body fat distribution and the metabolic complications of obesity. *J Clin Endocrinol Metab* **93**, S57-63 (2008).

198. Jialal, I., Devaraj, S., Kaur, H., Adams-Huet, B. & Bremer, A.A. Increased chemerin and decreased omentin-1 in both adipose tissue and plasma in nascent metabolic syndrome. *J Clin Endocrinol Metab* **98**, E514-517 (2013).

199. Voulgari, C., *et al.* Increased heart failure risk in normal-weight people with metabolic syndrome compared with metabolically healthy obese individuals. *J Am Coll Cardiol* **58**, 1343-1350 (2011).

200. Metric Views. Prospects improve for food energy labelling using SI units. (http://metricviews.org.uk/2012/02/prospects-improve-for-food-energy-labelling-using-si-units/, 2012).

201. Malik, V.S., Pan, A., Willett, W.C. & Hu, F.B. Sugar-sweetened beverages and weight gain in children and adults: a systematic review and meta-analysis. *Am J Clin Nutr* **98**, 1084-1102 (2013).

202. Phillips, C.M., *et al.* High dietary saturated fat intake accentuates obesity risk associated with the fat mass and obesity-associated gene in adults. *J Nutr* **142**, 824-831 (2012).

203. Bhutani, S. & Varady, K.A. Nibbling versus feasting: which meal pattern is better for heart disease prevention? *Nutrition reviews* **67**, 591-598 (2009).

204. Odegaard, A.O., *et al.* Breakfast frequency and development of metabolic risk. *Diabetes Care* **36**, 3100-3106 (2013).

205. Allison, K.C., Grilo, C.M., Masheb, R.M. & Stunkard, A.J. Binge eating disorder and night eating syndrome: a comparative study of disordered eating. *Journal of consulting and clinical psychology* **73**, 1107-1115 (2005).

206. WHO. Physical Activity and Adults. Recommended levels of physical activity for adults aged 18 - 64 years. (2011).

207. Maher, C.A., Mire, E., Harrington, D.M., Staiano, A.E. & Katzmarzyk, P.T. The independent and combined associations of physical activity and sedentary behavior with obesity in adults: NHANES 2003-06. *Obesity* **21**, E730-737 (2013).

208. Borghese, M.M., *et al.* Independent and combined associations of total sedentary time and television viewing time with food intake patterns of 9- to 11-year-old Canadian children. *Applied physiology, nutrition, and metabolism = Physiologie appliquee, nutrition et metabolisme* **39**, 937-943 (2014).

209. Bellisle, F. Meals and snacking, diet quality and energy balance. *Physiology & behavior* **134**, 38-43 (2014).

210. Patel, S.R. & Hu, F.B. Short sleep duration and weight gain: a systematic review. *Obesity* **16**, 643-653 (2008).

211. Nedeltcheva, A.V., Kilkus, J.M., Imperial, J., Schoeller, D.A. & Penev, P.D. Insufficient sleep undermines dietary efforts to reduce adiposity. *Ann Intern Med* **153**, 435-441 (2010).

212. Kalra, S.P., Bagnasco, M., Otukonyong, E.E., Dube, M.G. & Kalra, P.S. Rhythmic, reciprocal ghrelin and leptin signaling: new insight in the development of obesity. *Regulatory peptides* **111**, 1-11 (2003).

213. Spiegel, K., Tasali, E., Penev, P. & Van Cauter, E. Brief communication: Sleep

curtailment in healthy young men is associated with decreased leptin levels, elevated ghrelin levels, and increased hunger and appetite. *Ann Intern Med* **141**, 846-850 (2004).

214. Taheri, S., Lin, L., Austin, D., Young, T. & Mignot, E. Short sleep duration is associated with reduced leptin, elevated ghrelin, and increased body mass index. *PLoS medicine* **1**, e62 (2004).

215. Bouchard, C. Genetic determinants of regional fat distribution. *Hum Reprod* **12 Suppl 1**, 1-5 (1997).

216. Speiser, P.W., *et al.* Childhood obesity. *J Clin Endocrinol Metab* **90**, 1871-1887 (2005).

217. Reinehr, T., *et al.* Definable somatic disorders in overweight children and adolescents. *J Pediatr* **150**, 618-622, 622 e611-615 (2007).

218. Vaisse, C., *et al.* Melanocortin-4 receptor mutations are a frequent and heterogeneous cause of morbid obesity. *The Journal of clinical investigation* **106**, 253-262 (2000).

219. Dubern, B., *et al.* Homozygous null mutation of the melanocortin-4 receptor and severe early-onset obesity. *J Pediatr* **150**, 613-617, 617 e611 (2007).

220. Wolf, K.J. & Lorenz, R.G. Gut Microbiota and Obesity. *Current obesity reports* **1**, 1-8 (2012).

221. Liou, A.P., *et al.* Conserved shifts in the gut microbiota due to gastric bypass reduce host weight and adiposity. *Science translational medicine* **5**, 178ra141 (2013).

222. Ryan, K.K., *et al.* FXR is a molecular target for the effects of vertical sleeve gastrectomy. *Nature* **509**, 183-188 (2014).

223. Shen, J., Obin, M.S. & Zhao, L. The gut microbiota, obesity and insulin resistance. *Mol Aspects Med* **34**, 39-58 (2013).

224. Goodrich, J.K., *et al.* Human genetics shape the gut microbiome. *Cell* **159**, 789-799 (2014).

225. Pasarica, M., *et al.* Human adenovirus 36 induces adiposity, increases insulin sensitivity, and alters hypothalamic monoamines in rats. *Obesity* **14**, 1905-1913 (2006).

226. Angelakis, E., Armougom, F., Million, M. & Raoult, D. The relationship between gut microbiota and weight gain in humans. *Future microbiology* **7**, 91-109 (2012).

227. Backhed, F., *et al.* The gut microbiota as an environmental factor that regulates fat storage. *Proc Natl Acad Sci U S A* **101**, 15718-15723 (2004).

228. DiBaise, J.K., *et al.* Gut microbiota and its possible relationship with obesity. Mayo Clinic proceedings. *Mayo Clinic* **83**, 460-469 (2008).

229. Kalliomaki, M., Collado, M.C., Salminen, S. & Isolauri, E. Early differences in fecal microbiota composition in children may predict overweight. *Am J Clin Nutr* **87**, 534-538 (2008).

230. Cho, I., *et al.* Antibiotics in early life alter the murine colonic microbiome and adiposity. *Nature* **488**, 621-626 (2012).

231. Trasande, L., *et al.* Infant antibiotic exposures and early-life body mass. International journal of *obesity* **37**, 16-23 (2013).

232. Turnbaugh, P.J., *et al.* An obesity-associated gut microbiome with increased capacity for energy harvest. *Nature* **444**, 1027-1031 (2006).

233. Schecter, A., *et al.* Bisphenol A (BPA) in U.S. food. *Environ Sci Technol* **44**, 9425-9430 (2010).

234. Calafat, A.M., Ye, X., Wong, L.Y., Reidy, J.A. & Needham, L.L. Exposure of the

U.S. population to bisphenol A and 4-tertiary-octylphenol: 2003-2004. *Environ Health Perspect* **116**, 39-44 (2008).

235. Carwile, J.L. & Michels, K.B. Urinary bisphenol A and obesity: NHANES 2003-2006. *Environmental research* **111**, 825-830 (2011).

236. Lang, I.A., *et al.* Association of urinary bisphenol A concentration with medical disorders and laboratory abnormalities in adults. *JAMA* **300**, 1303-1310 (2008).

237. Melzer, D., *et al.* Urinary bisphenol A concentration and risk of future coronary artery disease in apparently healthy men and women. *Circulation* **125**, 1482-1490 (2012).

238. Trasande, L., Attina, T.M. & Blustein, J. Association between urinary bisphenol A concentration and obesity prevalence in children and adolescents. *JAMA* **308**, 1113-1121 (2012).

239. Takai, Y., *et al.* Preimplantation exposure to bisphenol A advances postnatal development. *Reproductive toxicology* **15**, 71-74 (2001).

240. Somm, E., *et al.* Perinatal exposure to bisphenol a alters early adipogenesis in the rat. *Environ Health Perspect* **117**, 1549-1555 (2009).

241. Vom Saal, F.S., Nagel, S.C., Coe, B.L., Angle, B.M. & Taylor, J.A. The estrogenic endocrine disrupting chemical bisphenol A (BPA) and obesity. *Mol Cell Endocrinol* **354**, 74-84 (2012).

242. Wardle, J., Carnell, S., Haworth, C.M. & Plomin, R. Evidence for a strong genetic influence on childhood adiposity despite the force of the obesogenic environment. *Am J Clin Nutr* **87**, 398-404 (2008).

243. Perusse, L., *et al.* The human obesity gene map: the 2004 update. *Obes Res* **13**, 381-490 (2005).

244. Stunkard, A.J., Harris, J.R., Pedersen, N.L. & McClearn, G.E. The body-mass index of twins who have been reared apart. *N Engl J Med* **322**, 1483-1487 (1990).

245. Maes, H.H., Neale, M.C. & Eaves, L.J. Genetic and environmental factors in relative body weight and human adiposity. *Behavior genetics* **27**, 325-351 (1997).

246. Rankinen, T., *et al.* The human obesity gene map: the 2001 update. *Obes Res* **10**, 196-243 (2002).

247. Cassidy, S.B., Schwartz, S., Miller, J.L. & Driscoll, D.J. Prader-Willi syndrome. *Genetics in medicine : official journal of the American College of Medical Genetics* **14**, 10-26 (2012).

248. Grace, C., *et al.* Energy metabolism in Bardet-Biedl syndrome. *International journal of obesity and related metabolic disorders : journal of the International Association for the Study of Obesity* **27**, 1319-1324 (2003).

249. Cassidy, S.B. & Driscoll, D.J. Prader-Willi syndrome. *European journal of human genetics : EJHG* **17**, 3-13 (2009).

250. Bonaglia, M.C., *et al.* Detailed phenotype-genotype study in five patients with chromosome 6q16 deletion: narrowing the critical region for Prader-Willi-like phenotype. *European journal of human genetics : EJHG* **16**, 1443-1449 (2008).

251. Crino, A., *et al.* Hypogonadism and pubertal development in Prader-Willi syndrome. *Eur J Pediatr* **162**, 327-333 (2003).

252. Butler, M.G. Management of obesity in Prader-Willi syndrome. *Nature clinical practice. Endocrinology & metabolism* **2**, 592-593 (2006).

253. Parfrey, P.S., Davidson, W.S. & Green, J.S. Clinical and genetic epidemiology of inherited renal disease in Newfoundland. *Kidney Int* **61**, 1925-1934 (2002).

254. Marion, V., *et al.* Transient ciliogenesis involving Bardet-Biedl syndrome proteins

is a fundamental characteristic of adipogenic differentiation. *Proc Natl Acad Sci U S A* **106**, 1820-1825 (2009).

255. Janssen, S., *et al*. Mutation analysis in Bardet-Biedl syndrome by DNA pooling and massively parallel resequencing in 105 individuals. *Hum Genet* **129**, 79-90 (2011).

256. Willer, C.J., *et al*. Six new loci associated with body mass index highlight a neuronal influence on body weight regulation. *Nat Genet* **41**, 25-34 (2009).

257. Frayling, T.M., *et al*. A common variant in the FTO gene is associated with body mass index and predisposes to childhood and adult obesity. *Science* **316**, 889-894 (2007).

258. Loos, R.J., *et al*. Common variants near MC4R are associated with fat mass, weight and risk of obesity. *Nat Genet* **40**, 768-775 (2008).

259. Speliotes, E.K., *et al*. Association analyses of 249,796 individuals reveal 18 new loci associated with body mass index. *Nat Genet* **42**, 937-948 (2010).

260. Thorleifsson, G., *et al*. Genome-wide association yields new sequence variants at seven loci that associate with measures of obesity. *Nat Genet* **41**, 18-24 (2009).

261. Bradfield, J.P., *et al*. A genome-wide association meta-analysis identifies new childhood obesity loci. *Nat Genet* **44**, 526-531 (2012).

262. Meyre, D., *et al*. Genome-wide association study for early-onset and morbid adult obesity identifies three new risk loci in European populations. *Nat Genet* **41**, 157-159 (2009).

263. Benzinou, M., *et al*. Common nonsynonymous variants in PCSK1 confer risk of obesity. *Nat Genet* **40**, 943-945 (2008).

264. Dina, C., *et al*. Variation in FTO contributes to childhood obesity and severe adult obesity. *Nat Genet* **39**, 724-726 (2007).

265. Han, J.C., *et al*. Brain-derived neurotrophic factor and obesity in the WAGR syndrome. *N Engl J Med* **359**, 918-927 (2008).

266. El-Gharbawy, A.H., *et al*. Serum brain-derived neurotrophic factor concentrations in lean and overweight children and adolescents. *J Clin Endocrinol Metab* **91**, 3548-3552 (2006).

267. Herbert, A., *et al*. A common genetic variant is associated with adult and childhood obesity. *Science* **312**, 279-283 (2006).

268. Lyon, H.N., *et al*. The association of a SNP upstream of INSIG2 with body mass index is reproduced in several but not all cohorts. *PLoS genetics* **3**, e61 (2007).

269. Ziouzenkova, O., *et al*. Retinaldehyde represses adipogenesis and diet-induced obesity. *Nature medicine* **13**, 695-702 (2007).

270. Troke, R.C., Tan, T.M. & Bloom, S.R. The future role of gut hormones in the treatment of obesity. *Therapeutic advances in chronic disease* **5**, 4-14 (2014).

271. Perry, B. & Wang, Y. Appetite regulation and weight control: the role of gut hormones. *Nutrition & diabetes* **2**, e26 (2012).

272. Suzuki, K., Jayasena, C.N. & Bloom, S.R. Obesity and appetite control. *Experimental diabetes research* **2012**, 824305 (2012).

273. Hagan, S. & Niswender, K.D. Neuroendocrine regulation of food intake. *Pediatr Blood Cancer* **58**, 149-153 (2012).

274. Murphy, K.G. & Bloom, S.R. Gut hormones in the control of appetite. *Experimental physiology* **89**, 507-516 (2004).

275. Small, C.J. & Bloom, S.R. Gut hormones and the control of appetite. *Trends in endocrinology and metabolism: TEM* **15**, 259-263 (2004).

276. Chaudhri, O.B., Wynne, K. & Bloom, S.R. Can gut hormones control appetite and prevent obesity? *Diabetes Care* **31** Suppl 2, S284-289 (2008).

277. Brennan, A.M. & Mantzoros, C.S. Drug Insight: the role of leptin in human physiology and pathophysiology--emerging clinical applications. Nature clinical practice. *Endocrinology & metabolism* **2**, 318-327 (2006).

278. Maffei, M., *et al*. Leptin levels in human and rodent: measurement of plasma leptin and ob RNA in obese and weight-reduced subjects. *Nature medicine* **1**, 1155-1161 (1995).

279. Considine, R.V. & Caro, J.F. Leptin in humans: current progress and future directions. *Clin Chem* **42**, 843-844 (1996).

280. Garcia-San Frutos, M., *et al*. Impaired central insulin response in aged Wistar rats: role of adiposity. *Endocrinology* **148**, 5238-5247 (2007).

281. Morrison, J.A., Glueck, C.J. & Wang, P. Preteen insulin levels interact with caloric intake to predict increases in obesity at ages 18 to 19 years: a 10-year prospective study of black and white girls. *Metabolism* **59**, 718-727 (2010).

282. Eu, C.H., Lim, W.Y., Ton, S.H. & bin Abdul Kadir, K. Glycyrrhizic acid improved lipoprotein lipase expression, insulin sensitivity, serum lipid and lipid deposition in high-fat diet-induced obese rats. *Lipids in health and disease* **9**, 81 (2010).

283. Kojima, M., *et al*. Ghrelin is a growth-hormone-releasing acylated peptide from stomach. *Nature* **402**, 656-660 (1999).

284. Hameed, S., Dhillo, W.S. & Bloom, S.R. Gut hormones and appetite control. *Oral diseases* **15**, 18-26 (2009).

285. Schwartz, M.W., Woods, S.C., Porte, D., Jr., Seeley, R.J. & Baskin, D.G. Central nervous system control of food intake. *Nature* **404**, 661-671 (2000).

286. Wren, A.M., *et al*. Ghrelin enhances appetite and increases food intake in humans. *J Clin Endocrinol Metab* **86**, 5992 (2001).

287. Druce, M.R., *et al*. Ghrelin increases food intake in obese as well as lean subjects. *International journal of obesity* **29**, 1130-1136 (2005).

288. Cummings, D.E., *et al*. Plasma ghrelin levels after diet-induced weight loss or gastric bypass surgery. *N Engl J Med* **346**, 1623-1630 (2002).

289. Perello, M., *et al*. Functional implications of limited leptin receptor and ghrelin receptor coexpression in the brain. *J Comp Neurol* **520**, 281-294 (2012).

290. Herrmann, C., *et al*. Glucagon-like peptide-1 and glucose-dependent insulin-releasing polypeptide plasma levels in response to nutrients. *Digestion* **56**, 117-126 (1995).

291. Marso, S.P., *et al*. Design of the liraglutide effect and action in diabetes: evaluation of cardiovascular outcome results (LEADER) trial. *Am Heart J* **166**, 823-830 e825 (2013).

292. Nauck, M., *et al*. Efficacy and safety comparison of liraglutide, glimepiride, and placebo, all in combination with metformin, in type 2 diabetes: the LEAD (liraglutide effect and action in diabetes)-2 study. *Diabetes Care* **32**, 84-90 (2009).

293. Vahl, T.P., Drazen, D.L., Seeley, R.J., D'Alessio, D.A. & Woods, S.C. Meal-anticipatory glucagon-like peptide-1 secretion in rats. *Endocrinology* **151**, 569-575 (2010).

294. Cummings, D.E. & Overduin, J. Gastrointestinal regulation of food intake. *The Journal of clinical investigation* **117**, 13-23 (2007).

295. Verdich, C., *et al*. A meta-analysis of the effect of glucagon-like peptide-1 (7-36) amide on ad libitum energy intake in humans. *J Clin Endocrinol Metab* **86**, 4382-

4389 (2001).

296. Gibbs, J., Young, R.C. & Smith, G.P. Cholecystokinin decreases food intake in rats. *Journal of comparative and physiological psychology* **84**, 488-495 (1973).

297. Buffa, R., Solcia, E. & Go, V.L. Immunohistochemical identification of the cholecystokinin cell in the intestinal mucosa. *Gastroenterology* **70**, 528-532 (1976).

298. Moran, T.H. & Schwartz, G.J. Neurobiology of cholecystokinin. *Critical reviews in neurobiology* **9**, 1-28 (1994).

299. Little, T.J., Horowitz, M. & Feinle-Bisset, C. Role of cholecystokinin in appetite control and body weight regulation. *Obesity reviews : an official journal of the International Association for the Study of Obesity* **6**, 297-306 (2005).

300. Batterham, R.L., *et al.* Pancreatic polypeptide reduces appetite and food intake in humans. *J Clin Endocrinol Metab* **88**, 3989-3992 (2003).

301. Malaisse-Lagae, F., Carpentier, J.L., Patel, Y.C., Malaisse, W.J. & Orci, L. Pancreatic polypeptide: a possible role in the regulation of food intake in the mouse. *Hypothesis. Experientia* **33**, 915-917 (1977).

302. Asakawa, A., *et al.* Characterization of the effects of pancreatic polypeptide in the regulation of energy balance. *Gastroenterology* **124**, 1325-1336 (2003).

303. Adrian, T.E., *et al.* Human distribution and release of a putative new gut hormone, peptide YY. *Gastroenterology* **89**, 1070-1077 (1985).

304. le Roux, C.W., *et al.* Attenuated peptide YY release in obese subjects is associated with reduced satiety. *Endocrinology* **147**, 3-8 (2006).

305. Alvarez Bartolome, M., *et al.* Peptide YY secretion in morbidly obese patients before and after vertical banded gastroplasty. *Obesity surgery* **12**, 324-327 (2002).

306. Murphy, K.G. & Bloom, S.R. Gut hormones and the regulation of energy homeostasis. *Nature* **444**, 854-859 (2006).

307. Batterham, R.L., *et al.* Inhibition of food intake in obese subjects by peptide YY3-36. *N Engl J Med* **349**, 941-948 (2003).

308. Druce, M.R. & Bloom, S.R. Oxyntomodulin : a novel potential treatment for obesity. *Treatments in endocrinology* **5**, 265-272 (2006).

309. Dakin, C.L., *et al.* Peripheral oxyntomodulin reduces food intake and body weight gain in rats. *Endocrinology* **145**, 2687-2695 (2004).

310. Holst, J.J. The physiology of glucagon-like peptide 1. *Physiol Rev* **87**, 1409-1439 (2007).

311. Pocai, A. Unraveling oxyntomodulin, GLP1's enigmatic brother. *J Endocrinol* **215**, 335-346 (2012).

312. Schjoldager, B., Mortensen, P.E., Myhre, J., Christiansen, J. & Holst, J.J. Oxyntomodulin from distal gut. Role in regulation of gastric and pancreatic functions. *Dig Dis Sci* **34**, 1411-1419 (1989).

313. Wynne, K., *et al.* Oxyntomodulin increases energy expenditure in addition to decreasing energy intake in overweight and obese humans: a randomised controlled trial. *International journal of obesity* **30**, 1729-1736 (2006).

314. Baggio, L.L., Huang, Q., Brown, T.J. & Drucker, D.J. Oxyntomodulin and glucagon-like peptide-1 differentially regulate murine food intake and energy expenditure. *Gastroenterology* **127**, 546-558 (2004).

315. Schjoldager, B.T., Baldissera, F.G., Mortensen, P.E., Holst, J.J. & Christiansen, J. Oxyntomodulin: a potential hormone from the distal gut. Pharmacokinetics and effects on gastric acid and insulin secretion in man. *Eur J Clin Invest* **18**, 499-503 (1988).

316. Kosinski, J.R., *et al.* The glucagon receptor is involved in mediating the body weight-lowering effects of oxyntomodulin. *Obesity* **20**, 1566-1571 (2012).
317. Kobelt, P., *et al.* Bombesin, but not amylin, blocks the orexigenic effect of peripheral ghrelin. *American journal of physiology. Regulatory, integrative and comparative physiology* **291**, R903-913 (2006).
318. Furutani, N., Hondo, M., Tsujino, N. & Sakurai, T. Activation of bombesin receptor subtype-3 influences activity of orexin neurons by both direct and indirect pathways. *Journal of molecular neuroscience : MN* **42**, 106-111 (2010).
319. Bays, H.E. Current and investigational antiobesity agents and obesity therapeutic treatment targets. *Obes Res* **12**, 1197-1211 (2004).
320. Crowley, V.E. Overview of human obesity and central mechanisms regulating energy homeostasis. *Annals of clinical biochemistry* **45**, 245-255 (2008).
321. Iglesias, P., Selgas, R., Romero, S. & Diez, J.J. Biological role, clinical significance, and therapeutic possibilities of the recently discovered metabolic hormone fibroblastic growth factor 21. *Eur J Endocrinol* **167**, 301-309 (2012).
322. Coskun, T. Fibroblast growth factor 21 (FGF21) increases energy expenditure in a leptin-dependent manner. in *48th Annaual Meeting of European Association for the Study of Diabetes (EASD)* (Berlin, Germany, 2013).
323. Persani, L. Clinical review: Central hypothyroidism: pathogenic, diagnostic, and therapeutic challenges. *J Clin Endocrinol Metab* **97**, 3068-3078 (2012).
324. Guyton, A.C. & Hall, J.E. *Textbook of Medical Physiology*, (Elsevier Inc., Philadelphia, 2006).
325. Sharma, S.T. & Nieman, L.K. Cushing's syndrome: all variants, detection, and treatment. *Endocrinol Metab Clin North Am* **40**, 379-391, viii-ix (2011).
326. Sacker, I.M. & Buff, S. *Regaining Your Self: Understanding and Conquering the Eating Disorder Identity*, (Health Communications, Inc., Deerfielsd Beach, Florida, USA 2010).
327. Licinio, J., *et al.* Phenotypic effects of leptin replacement on morbid obesity, diabetes mellitus, hypogonadism, and behavior in leptin-deficient adults. *Proc Natl Acad Sci U S A* **101**, 4531-4536 (2004).
328. Ramachandrappa, S. & Farooqi, I.S. Genetic approaches to understanding human obesity. *The Journal of clinical investigation* **121**, 2080-2086 (2011).
329. Liao, G.Y., *et al.* Dendritically targeted Bdnf mRNA is essential for energy balance and response to leptin. *Nature medicine* **18**, 564-571 (2012).
330. Kohlstadt, I. & Wharton, G. Clinician uptake of obesity-related drug information: a qualitative assessment using continuing medical education activities. *Nutrition journal* **12**, 44 (2013).
331. Mantzoros, C.S., *et al.* Cord blood leptin and adiponectin as predictors of adiposity in children at 3 years of age: a prospective cohort study. *Pediatrics* **123**, 682-689 (2009).
332. Chiavaroli, V., *et al.* Insulin resistance and oxidative stress in children born small and large for gestational age. *Pediatrics* **124**, 695-702 (2009).
333. Renom Espineira, A., *et al.* Postnatal growth and cardiometabolic profile in young adults born large for gestational age. *Clin Endocrinol (Oxf)* **75**, 335-341 (2011).
334. Efstathiou, S.P., Skeva, II, Zorbala, E., Georgiou, E. & Mountokalakis, T.D. Metabolic syndrome in adolescence: can it be predicted from natal and parental profile? The Prediction of Metabolic Syndrome in Adolescence (PREMA) study. *Circulation* **125**, 902-910 (2012).

335. Huxley, R., *et al.* Is birth weight a risk factor for ischemic heart disease in later life? *Am J Clin Nutr* **85**, 1244-1250 (2007).

336. Barker, D.J., Winter, P.D., Osmond, C., Margetts, B. & Simmonds, S.J. Weight in infancy and death from ischaemic heart disease. *Lancet* **2**, 577-580 (1989).

337. Fernandez-Twinn, D.S. & Ozanne, S.E. Mechanisms by which poor early growth programs type-2 diabetes, obesity and the metabolic syndrome. *Physiology & behavior* **88**, 234-243 (2006).

338. Plagemann, A. Perinatal nutrition and hormone-dependent programming of food intake. *Horm Res* **65 Suppl** 3, 83-89 (2006).

339. van Abeelen, A.F., *et al.* Survival effects of prenatal famine exposure. *Am J Clin Nutr* **95**, 179-183 (2012).

340. Ludwig, D.S. & Currie, J. The association between pregnancy weight gain and birthweight: a within-family comparison. *Lancet* **376**, 984-990 (2010).

341. Deierlein, A.L., Siega-Riz, A.M., Adair, L.S. & Herring, A.H. Effects of pre-pregnancy body mass index and gestational weight gain on infant anthropometric outcomes. *J Pediatr* **158**, 221-226 (2011).

342. Lawlor, D.A., Lichtenstein, P. & Langstrom, N. Association of maternal diabetes mellitus in pregnancy with offspring adiposity into early adulthood: sibling study in a prospective cohort of 280,866 men from 248,293 families. *Circulation* **123**, 258-265 (2011).

343. Davis, E.F., *et al.* Cardiovascular risk factors in children and young adults born to preeclamptic pregnancies: a systematic review. *Pediatrics* **129**, e1552-1561 (2012).

344. Washburn, L., Nixon, P., Russell, G., Snively, B.M. & O'Shea, T.M. Adiposity in adolescent offspring born prematurely to mothers with preeclampsia. *J Pediatr* **162**, 912-917 e911 (2013).

345. Seidman, D.S., *et al.* Pre-eclampsia and offspring's blood pressure, cognitive ability and physical development at 17-years-of-age. *Br J Obstet Gynaecol* **98**, 1009-1014 (1991).

346. Ogland, B., Vatten, L.J., Romundstad, P.R., Nilsen, S.T. & Forman, M.R. Pubertal anthropometry in sons and daughters of women with preeclamptic or normotensive pregnancies. *Arch Dis Child* **94**, 855-859 (2009).

347. Kral, J.G., *et al.* Large maternal weight loss from obesity surgery prevents transmission of obesity to children who were followed for 2 to 18 years. *Pediatrics* **118**, e1644-1649 (2006).

348. Taveras, E.M., *et al.* Weight status in the first 6 months of life and obesity at 3 years of age. *Pediatrics* **123**, 1177-1183 (2009).

349. Fraser, A., *et al.* Association of maternal weight gain in pregnancy with offspring obesity and metabolic and vascular traits in childhood. *Circulation* **121**, 2557-2564 (2010).

350. Taveras, E.M., *et al.* Crossing growth percentiles in infancy and risk of obesity in childhood. *Arch Pediatr Adolesc Med* **165**, 993-998 (2011).

351. Leunissen, R.W., Kerkhof, G.F., Stijnen, T. & Hokken-Koelega, A. Timing and tempo of first-year rapid growth in relation to cardiovascular and metabolic risk profile in early adulthood. *JAMA* **301**, 2234-2242 (2009).

352. Monteiro, P.O. & Victora, C.G. Rapid growth in infancy and childhood and obesity in later life--a systematic review. *Obesity reviews : an official journal of the International Association for the Study of Obesity* **6**, 143-154 (2005).

353. Ong, K.K. & Loos, R.J. Rapid infancy weight gain and subsequent obesity:

systematic reviews and hopeful suggestions. *Acta Paediatr* **95**, 904-908 (2006).

354. Owen, C.G., Martin, R.M., Whincup, P.H., Smith, G.D. & Cook, D.G. Effect of infant feeding on the risk of obesity across the life course: a quantitative review of published evidence. *Pediatrics* **115**, 1367-1377 (2005).

355. Baird, J., *et al.* Being big or growing fast: systematic review of size and growth in infancy and later obesity. *BMJ* **331**, 929 (2005).

356. Belfort, M.B., Rifas-Shiman, S.L., Rich-Edwards, J., Kleinman, K.P. & Gillman, M.W. Size at birth, infant growth, and blood pressure at three years of age. *J Pediatr* **151**, 670-674 (2007).

357. Shehadeh, N., Weitzer-Kish, H., Shamir, R., Shihab, S. & Weiss, R. Impact of early postnatal weight gain and feeding patterns on body mass index in adolescence. *J Pediatr Endocrinol Metab* **21**, 9-15 (2008).

358. Gardner, D.S., *et al.* Contribution of early weight gain to childhood overweight and metabolic health: a longitudinal study (EarlyBird 36). *Pediatrics* **123**, e67-73 (2009).

359. Skilton, M.R., *et al.* Weight gain in infancy and vascular risk factors in later childhood. *Pediatrics* **131**, e1821-1828 (2013).

360. Yeung, M.Y. Postnatal growth, neurodevelopment and altered adiposity after preterm birth--from a clinical nutrition perspective. *Acta Paediatr* **95**, 909-917 (2006).

361. Lucas, A., Morley, R. & Cole, T.J. Randomised trial of early diet in preterm babies and later intelligence quotient. *BMJ* **317**, 1481-1487 (1998).

362. Thureen, P.J. The neonatologist's dilemma: catch-up growth or beneficial undernutrition in very low birth weight infants-what are optimal growth rates? *Journal of pediatric gastroenterology and nutrition* **45 Suppl 3**, S152-154 (2007).

363. Kerkhof, G.F., Willemsen, R.H., Leunissen, R.W., Breukhoven, P.E. & Hokken-Koelega, A.C. Health profile of young adults born preterm: negative effects of rapid weight gain in early life. *J Clin Endocrinol Metab* **97**, 4498-4506 (2012).

364. Ong, K.K., *et al.* Earlier mother's age at menarche predicts rapid infancy growth and childhood obesity. *PLoS medicine* **4**, e132 (2007).

365. Davey Smith, G., Steer, C., Leary, S. & Ness, A. Is there an intrauterine influence on obesity? Evidence from parent child associations in the Avon Longitudinal Study of Parents and Children (ALSPAC). *Arch Dis Child* **92**, 876-880 (2007).

366. Onyike, C.U., Crum, R.M., Lee, H.B., Lyketsos, C.G. & Eaton, W.W. Is obesity associated with major depression? Results from the Third National Health and Nutrition Examination Survey. *Am J Epidemiol* **158**, 1139-1147 (2003).

367. Levitan, R.D., *et al.* The dopamine-4 receptor gene associated with binge eating and weight gain in women with seasonal affective disorder: an evolutionary perspective. *Biol Psychiatry* **56**, 665-669 (2004).

368. Unger, R., Kreeger, L. & Christoffel, K.K. Childhood obesity. Medical and familial correlates and age of onset. *Clin Pediatr (Phila)* **29**, 368-373 (1990).

369. van Dam, R.M., Willett, W.C., Manson, J.E. & Hu, F.B. The relationship between overweight in adolescence and premature death in women. *Ann Intern Med* **145**, 91-97 (2006).

370. Must, A., Jacques, P.F., Dallal, G.E., Bajema, C.J. & Dietz, W.H. Long-term morbidity and mortality of overweight adolescents. A follow-up of the Harvard Growth Study of 1922 to 1935. *N Engl J Med* **327**, 1350-1355 (1992).

371. Bjorge, T., Engeland, A., Tverdal, A. & Smith, G.D. Body mass index in

adolescence in relation to cause-specific mortality: a follow-up of 230,000 Norwegian adolescents. *Am J Epidemiol* **168**, 30-37 (2008).

372. Williams, D.E., *et al.* Prevalence of impaired fasting glucose and its relationship with cardiovascular disease risk factors in US adolescents, 1999-2000. *Pediatrics* **116**, 1122-1126 (2005).

373. Sabin, M.A., *et al.* Characterisation of morbidity in a UK, hospital based, obesity clinic. *Arch Dis Child* **91**, 126-130 (2006).

374. Healthy Study Group, *et al.* Risk factors for type 2 diabetes in a sixth- grade multiracial cohort: the HEALTHY study. Diabetes Care 32, 953-955 (2009).

375. Marcus, M.D., *et al.* Severe obesity and selected risk factors in a sixth grade multiracial cohort: the HEALTHY study. *The Journal of adolescent health : official publication of the Society for Adolescent Medicine* **47**, 604-607 (2010).

376. Sinha, R., *et al.* Prevalence of impaired glucose tolerance among children and adolescents with marked obesity. *N Engl J Med* **346**, 802-810 (2002).

377. Shalitin, S., Abrahami, M., Lilos, P. & Phillip, M. Insulin resistance and impaired glucose tolerance in obese children and adolescents referred to a tertiary-care center in Israel. *International journal of obesity* **29**, 571-578 (2005).

378. Maffeis, C., *et al.* Fasting plasma glucose (FPG) and the risk of impaired glucose tolerance in obese children and adolescents. *Obesity* **18**, 1437-1442 (2010).

379. Shah, S., Kublaoui, B.M., Oden, J.D. & White, P.C. Screening for type 2 diabetes in obese youth. *Pediatrics* **124**, 573-579 (2009).

380. Keskin, M., Kurtoglu, S., Kendirci, M., Atabek, M.E. & Yazici, C. Homeostasis model assessment is more reliable than the fasting glucose/insulin ratio and quantitative insulin sensitivity check index for assessing insulin resistance among obese children and adolescents. *Pediatrics* **115**, e500-503 (2005).

381. Moller, D.E. & Flier, J.S. Insulin resistance--mechanisms, syndromes, and implications. *N Engl J Med* **325**, 938-948 (1991).

382. Matthews, D.R., *et al.* Homeostasis model assessment: insulin resistance and beta-cell function from fasting plasma glucose and insulin concentrations in man. *Diabetologia* **28**, 412-419 (1985).

383. Silfen, M.E., *et al.* Comparison of simple measures of insulin sensitivity in young girls with premature adrenarche: the fasting glucose to insulin ratio may be a simple and useful measure. *J Clin Endocrinol Metab* **86**, 2863-2868 (2001).

384. Vuguin, P., Saenger, P. & Dimartino-Nardi, J. Fasting glucose insulin ratio: a useful measure of insulin resistance in girls with premature adrenarche. *J Clin Endocrinol Metab* **86**, 4618-4621 (2001).

385. Dimartino-Nardi, J. Premature adrenarche: findings in prepubertal African-American and Caribbean-Hispanic girls. *Acta Paediatr Suppl* **88**, 67-72 (1999).

386. Katz, A., *et al.* Quantitative insulin sensitivity check index: a simple, accurate method for assessing insulin sensitivity in humans. *J Clin Endocrinol Metab* **85**, 2402-2410 (2000).

387. Buchanan, T.A., Watanabe, R.M. & Xiang, A.H. Limitations in surrogate measures of insulin resistance. *J Clin Endocrinol Metab* **95**, 4874-4876 (2010).

388. Conwell, L.S., Trost, S.G., Brown, W.J. & Batch, J.A. Indexes of insulin resistance and secretion in obese children and adolescents: a validation study. *Diabetes Care* **27**, 314-319 (2004).

389. Brandou, F., Brun, J.F. & Mercier, J. Limited accuracy of surrogates of insulin resistance during puberty in obese and lean children at risk for altered

glucoregulation. *J Clin Endocrinol Metab* **90**, 761-767 (2005).

390. Uwaifo, G.I., *et al.* Indices of insulin action, disposal, and secretion derived from fasting samples and clamps in normal glucose-tolerant black and white children. *Diabetes Care* **25**, 2081-2087 (2002).

391. Gungor, N., Saad, R., Janosky, J. & Arslanian, S. Validation of surrogate estimates of insulin sensitivity and insulin secretion in children and adolescents. *J Pediatr* **144**, 47-55 (2004).

392. Muniyappa, R., Lee, S., Chen, H. & Quon, M.J. Current approaches for assessing insulin sensitivity and resistance in vivo: advantages, limitations, and appropriate usage. *Am J Physiol Endocrinol Metab* **294**, E15-26 (2008).

393. Sjaarda, L.G., *et al.* Oral disposition index in obese youth from normal to prediabetes to diabetes: relationship to clamp disposition index. *J Pediatr* **161**, 51-57 (2012).

394. American Diabetes, A. Standards of medical care in diabetes--2010. *Diabetes Care* **33 Suppl 1**, S11-61 (2010).

395. Molnar, D. The prevalence of the metabolic syndrome and type 2 diabetes mellitus in children and adolescents. *International journal of obesity and related metabolic disorders : journal of the International Association for the Study of Obesity* **28 Suppl 3**, S70-74 (2004).

396. Pinhas-Hamiel, O., *et al.* Increased incidence of non-insulin-dependent diabetes mellitus among adolescents. *J Pediatr* **128**, 608-615 (1996).

397. Goran, M.I., *et al.* Low prevalence of pediatric type 2 diabetes: where's the epidemic? *J Pediatr* **152**, 753-755 (2008).

398. Hannon, T.S., Rao, G. & Arslanian, S.A. Childhood obesity and type 2 diabetes mellitus. *Pediatrics* **116**, 473-480 (2005).

399. Copeland, K.C., *et al.* Characteristics of adolescents and youth with recent-onset type 2 diabetes: the TODAY cohort at baseline. *J Clin Endocrinol Metab* **96**, 159-167 (2011).

400. Tirosh, A., *et al.* Adolescent BMI trajectory and risk of diabetes versus coronary disease. *N Engl J Med* **364**, 1315-1325 (2011).

401. Gallagher, E.J., Leroith, D. & Karnieli, E. The metabolic syndrome--from insulin resistance to obesity and diabetes. *The Medical clinics of North America* **95**, 855-873 (2011).

402. Steinberger, J., *et al.* Progress and challenges in metabolic syndrome in children and adolescents: a scientific statement from the American Heart Association Atherosclerosis, Hypertension, and Obesity in the Young Committee of the Council on Cardiovascular Disease in the Young; Council on Cardiovascular Nursing; and Council on Nutrition, Physical Activity, and Metabolism. *Circulation* **119**, 628-647 (2009).

403. Weiss, R., *et al.* Obesity and the metabolic syndrome in children and adolescents. *N Engl J Med* **350**, 2362-2374 (2004).

404. Cook, S., Weitzman, M., Auinger, P., Nguyen, M. & Dietz, W.H. Prevalence of a metabolic syndrome phenotype in adolescents: findings from the third National Health and Nutrition Examination Survey, 1988-1994. *Arch Pediatr Adolesc Med* **157**, 821-827 (2003).

405. Lambert, M., *et al.* Insulin resistance syndrome in a representative sample of children and adolescents from Quebec, Canada. *International journal of obesity and related metabolic disorders : journal of the International Association for the Study of*

Obesity **28**, 833-841 (2004).

406. Goodman, E., Daniels, S.R., Meigs, J.B. & Dolan, L.M. Instability in the diagnosis of metabolic syndrome in adolescents. *Circulation* **115**, 2316-2322 (2007).

407. Chi, C.H., Wang, Y., Wilson, D.M. & Robinson, T.N. Definition of metabolic syndrome in preadolescent girls. *J Pediatr* **148**, 788-792 (2006).

408. Zimmet, P., *et al.* The metabolic syndrome in children and adolescents. *Lancet* **369**, 2059-2061 (2007).

409. Garn, S.M. & Clark, D.C. Nutrition, growth, development, and maturation: findings from the ten-state nutrition survey of 1968-1970. *Pediatrics* **56**, 306-319 (1975).

410. Laron, Z. Is obesity associated with early sexual maturation? *Pediatrics* **113**, 171-172; author reply 171-172 (2004).

411. Wang, Y. Is obesity associated with early sexual maturation? A comparison of the association in American boys versus girls. *Pediatrics* **110**, 903-910 (2002).

412. Kaplowitz, P.B., Slora, E.J., Wasserman, R.C., Pedlow, S.E. & Herman-Giddens, M.E. Earlier onset of puberty in girls: relation to increased body mass index and race. *Pediatrics* **108**, 347-353 (2001).

413. Herman-Giddens, M.E., *et al.* Secondary sexual characteristics in boys: data from the Pediatric Research in Office Settings Network. *Pediatrics* **130**, e1058-1068 (2012).

414. Halpern, A., *et al.* Metabolic syndrome, dyslipidemia, hypertension and type 2 diabetes in youth: from diagnosis to treatment. *Diabetology & metabolic syndrome* **2**, 55 (2010).

415. Li, S., Chen, W., Srinivasan, S.R., Xu, J. & Berenson, G.S. Relation of childhood obesity/cardiometabolic phenotypes to adult cardiometabolic profile: the Bogalusa Heart Study. *Am J Epidemiol* **176 Suppl** 7, S142-149 (2012).

416. Friedemann, C., *et al.* Cardiovascular disease risk in healthy children and its association with body mass index: systematic review and meta-analysis. *BMJ* **345**, e4759 (2012).

417. Sorof, J. & Daniels, S. Obesity hypertension in children: a problem of epidemic proportions. *Hypertension* **40**, 441-447 (2002).

418. Maggio, A.B., *et al.* Associations among obesity, blood pressure, and left ventricular mass. *J Pediatr* **152**, 489-493 (2008).

419. Stabouli, S., Kotsis, V., Papamichael, C., Constantopoulos, A. & Zakopoulos, N. Adolescent obesity is associated with high ambulatory blood pressure and increased carotid intimal-medial thickness. *J Pediatr* **147**, 651-656 (2005).

420. Aguilar, A., Ostrow, V., De Luca, F. & Suarez, E. Elevated ambulatory blood pressure in a multi-ethnic population of obese children and adolescents. *J Pediatr* **156**, 930-935 (2010).

421. O'Brien, E., *et al.* European Society of Hypertension position paper on ambulatory blood pressure monitoring. *J Hypertens* **31**, 1731-1768 (2013).

422. Hanevold, C., *et al.* The effects of obesity, gender, and ethnic group on left ventricular hypertrophy and geometry in hypertensive children: a collaborative study of the International Pediatric Hypertension Association. *Pediatrics* **113**, 328-333 (2004).

423. Urbina, E.M., Gidding, S.S., Bao, W., Elkasabany, A. & Berenson, G.S. Association of fasting blood sugar level, insulin level, and obesity with left ventricular mass in healthy children and adolescents: The Bogalusa Heart Study.

Am Heart J **138**, 122-127 (1999).

424. Urbina, E.M., *et al.* Effect of body size, ponderosity, and blood pressure on left ventricular growth in children and young adults in the Bogalusa Heart Study. *Circulation* **91**, 2400-2406 (1995).

425. Chinali, M., *et al.* Impact of obesity on cardiac geometry and function in a population of adolescents: the Strong Heart Study. *J Am Coll Cardiol* **47**, 2267-2273 (2006).

426. Crowley, D.I., Khoury, P.R., Urbina, E.M., Ippisch, H.M. & Kimball, T.R. Cardiovascular impact of the pediatric obesity epidemic: higher left ventricular mass is related to higher body mass index. *J Pediatr* **158**, 709-714 e701 (2011).

427. Sun, S.S., *et al.* Systolic blood pressure in childhood predicts hypertension and metabolic syndrome later in life. *Pediatrics* **119**, 237-246 (2007).

428. Dietz, W.H. Health consequences of obesity in youth: childhood predictors of adult disease. *Pediatrics* **101**, 518-525 (1998).

429. Williams, D.P., *et al.* Body fatness and risk for elevated blood pressure, total cholesterol, and serum lipoprotein ratios in children and adolescents. *American journal of public health* **82**, 358-363 (1992).

430. Harel, Z., Riggs, S., Vaz, R., Flanagan, P. & Harel, D. Isolated low HDL cholesterol emerges as the most common lipid abnormality among obese adolescents. *Clin Pediatr (Phila)* **49**, 29-34 (2010).

431. Morrison, J.A., Sprecher, D.L., Barton, B.A., Waclawiw, M.A. & Daniels, S.R. Overweight, fat patterning, and cardiovascular disease risk factors in black and white girls: The National Heart, Lung, and Blood Institute Growth and Health Study. *J Pediatr* **135**, 458-464 (1999).

432. Caprio, S., *et al.* Fat distribution and cardiovascular risk factors in obese adolescent girls: importance of the intraabdominal fat depot. *Am J Clin Nutr* **64**, 12-17 (1996).

433. Freedman, D.S., *et al.* The relation of obesity throughout life to carotid intima-media thickness in adulthood: the Bogalusa Heart Study. *International journal of obesity and related metabolic disorders : journal of the International Association for the Study of Obesity* **28**, 159-166 (2004).

434. Tounian, P., *et al.* Presence of increased stiffness of the common carotid artery and endothelial dysfunction in severely obese children: a prospective study. *Lancet* **358**, 1400-1404 (2001).

435. Zhu, W., Huang, X., He, J., Li, M. & Neubauer, H. Arterial intima-media thickening and endothelial dysfunction in obese Chinese children. *Eur J Pediatr* **164**, 337-344 (2005).

436. Woo, K.S., *et al.* Overweight in children is associated with arterial endothelial dysfunction and intima-media thickening. *International journal of obesity and related metabolic disorders : journal of the International Association for the Study of Obesity* **28**, 852-857 (2004).

437. Whincup, P.H., *et al.* Arterial distensibility in adolescents: the influence of adiposity, the metabolic syndrome, and classic risk factors. *Circulation* **112**, 1789-1797 (2005).

438. Iannuzzi, A., *et al.* Increased carotid intima-media thickness and stiffness in obese children. *Diabetes Care* **27**, 2506-2508 (2004).

439. Yu, J.J., Yeom, H.H., Chung, S., Park, Y. & Lee, D.H. Left atrial diameters in overweight children with normal blood pressure. *J Pediatr* **148**, 321-325 (2006).

440. Meyer, A.A., Kundt, G., Steiner, M., Schuff-Werner, P. & Kienast, W. Impaired flow-mediated vasodilation, carotid artery intima-media thickening, and elevated endothelial plasma markers in obese children: the impact of cardiovascular risk factors. *Pediatrics* **117**, 1560-1567 (2006).

441. Groner, J.A., Joshi, M. & Bauer, J.A. Pediatric precursors of adult cardiovascular disease: noninvasive assessment of early vascular changes in children and adolescents. *Pediatrics* **118**, 1683-1691 (2006).

442. Mittelman, S.D., *et al.* Adiposity predicts carotid intima-media thickness in healthy children and adolescents. *J Pediatr* **156**, 592-597 e592 (2010).

443. Skinner, A.C., Steiner, M.J., Henderson, F.W. & Perrin, E.M. Multiple markers of inflammation and weight status: cross-sectional analyses throughout childhood. *Pediatrics* **125**, e801-809 (2010).

444. Osiniri, I., *et al.* Carotid intima-media thickness at 7 years of age: relationship to C-reactive protein rather than adiposity. *J Pediatr* **160**, 276-280 e271 (2012).

445. Atabek, M.E., Pirgon, O. & Kivrak, A.S. Evidence for association between insulin resistance and premature carotid atherosclerosis in childhood obesity. *Pediatr Res* **61**, 345-349 (2007).

446. Zhu, H., *et al.* Relationships of cardiovascular phenotypes with healthy weight, at risk of overweight, and overweight in US youths. *Pediatrics* **121**, 115-122 (2008).

447. Baker, J.L., Olsen, L.W. & Sorensen, T.I. Childhood body-mass index and the risk of coronary heart disease in adulthood. *N Engl J Med* **357**, 2329-2337 (2007).

448. Bibbins-Domingo, K., Coxson, P., Pletcher, M.J., Lightwood, J. & Goldman, L. Adolescent overweight and future adult coronary heart disease. *N Engl J Med* **357**, 2371-2379 (2007).

449. Haslam, D.W. & James, W.P. Obesity. *Lancet* **366**, 1197-1209 (2005).

450. Kurth, T., *et al.* Prospective study of body mass index and risk of stroke in apparently healthy women. *Circulation* **111**, 1992-1998 (2005).

451. Kurth, T., *et al.* Body mass index and the risk of stroke in men. *Arch Intern Med* **162**, 2557-2562 (2002).

452. Bigal, M.E. & Lipton, R.B. Obesity and chronic daily headache. *Current pain and headache reports* **12**, 56-61 (2008).

453. Peres, M.F., Lerario, D.D., Garrido, A.B. & Zukerman, E. Primary headaches in obese patients. *Arquivos de neuro-psiquiatria* **63**, 931-933 (2005).

454. Matteoni, C.A., *et al.* Nonalcoholic fatty liver disease: a spectrum of clinical and pathological severity. *Gastroenterology* **116**, 1413-1419 (1999).

455. Lavine, J.E. & Schwimmer, J.B. Nonalcoholic fatty liver disease in the pediatric population. *Clin Liver Dis* **8**, 549-558, viii-ix (2004).

456. Huang, J.S., *et al.* Childhood obesity for pediatric gastroenterologists. *Journal of pediatric gastroenterology and nutrition* **56**, 99-109 (2013).

457. Feldstein, A.E., *et al.* The natural history of non-alcoholic fatty liver disease in children: a follow-up study for up to 20 years. *Gut* **58**, 1538-1544 (2009).

458. Mandato, C., *et al.* Metabolic, hormonal, oxidative, and inflammatory factors in pediatric obesity-related liver disease. *J Pediatr* **147**, 62-66 (2005).

459. Schwimmer, J.B., *et al.* Obesity, insulin resistance, and other clinicopathological correlates of pediatric nonalcoholic fatty liver disease. *J Pediatr* **143**, 500-505 (2003).

460. Schwimmer, J.B., Pardee, P.E., Lavine, J.E., Blumkin, A.K. & Cook, S. Cardiovascular risk factors and the metabolic syndrome in pediatric nonalcoholic

fatty liver disease. *Circulation* **118**, 277-283 (2008).

461. Strauss, R.S., Barlow, S.E. & Dietz, W.H. Prevalence of abnormal serum aminotransferase values in overweight and obese adolescents. *J Pediatr* **136**, 727-733 (2000).

462. Schwimmer, J.B., McGreal, N., Deutsch, R., Finegold, M.J. & Lavine, J.E. Influence of gender, race, and ethnicity on suspected fatty liver in obese adolescents. *Pediatrics* **115**, e561-565 (2005).

463. Welsh, J.A., Karpen, S. & Vos, M.B. Increasing prevalence of nonalcoholic fatty liver disease among United States adolescents, 1988-1994 to 2007-2010. *J Pediatr* **162**, 496-500 e491 (2013).

464. Schwimmer, J.B., *et al.* Prevalence of fatty liver in children and adolescents. *Pediatrics* **118**, 1388-1393 (2006).

465. Tominaga, K., *et al.* Prevalence of fatty liver in Japanese children and relationship to obesity. An epidemiological ultrasonographic survey. *Dig Dis Sci* **40**, 2002-2009 (1995).

466. Chan, D.F., *et al.* Hepatic steatosis in obese Chinese children. *International journal of obesity and related metabolic disorders : journal of the International Association for the Study of Obesity* **28**, 1257-1263 (2004).

467. Baldridge, A.D., Perez-Atayde, A.R., Graeme-Cook, F., Higgins, L. & Lavine, J.E. Idiopathic steatohepatitis in childhood: a multicenter retrospective study. *J Pediatr* **127**, 700-704 (1995).

468. Franzese, A., *et al.* Liver involvement in obese children. Ultrasonography and liver enzyme levels at diagnosis and during follow-up in an Italian population. *Dig Dis Sci* **42**, 1428-1432 (1997).

469. Tazawa, Y., Noguchi, H., Nishinomiya, F. & Takada, G. Serum alanine aminotransferase activity in obese children. *Acta Paediatr* **86**, 238-241 (1997).

470. Kinugasa, A., *et al.* Fatty liver and its fibrous changes found in simple obesity of children. *Journal of pediatric gastroenterology and nutrition* **3**, 408-414 (1984).

471. Huang, J.S., *et al.* Consensus Statement: Childhood Obesity for Pediatric Gastroenterologists. *Journal of pediatric gastroenterology and nutrition* (2012).

472. Radetti, G., Kleon, W., Stuefer, J. & Pittschieler, K. Non-alcoholic fatty liver disease in obese children evaluated by magnetic resonance imaging. *Acta Paediatr* **95**, 833-837 (2006).

473. Shannon, A., *et al.* Ultrasonographic quantitative estimation of hepatic steatosis in children With NAFLD. *Journal of pediatric gastroenterology and nutrition* **53**, 190-195 (2011).

474. Vajro, P., *et al.* Persistent hyperaminotransferasemia resolving after weight reduction in obese children. *J Pediatr* **125**, 239-241 (1994).

475. Rashid, M. & Roberts, E.A. Nonalcoholic steatohepatitis in children. *Journal of pediatric gastroenterology and nutrition* **30**, 48-53 (2000).

476. McNair, A. Non-alcoholic steatohepatitis (NASH): why biopsy? *Gut* **51**, 898; author reply 898-899 (2002).

477. Bohte, A.E., *et al.* US cannot be used to predict the presence or severity of hepatic steatosis in severely obese adolescents. *Radiology* **262**, 327-334 (2012).

478. Huang, M.A., *et al.* One-year intense nutritional counseling results in histological improvement in patients with non-alcoholic steatohepatitis: a pilot study. *The American journal of gastroenterology* **100**, 1072-1081 (2005).

479. Reinehr, T., Schmidt, C., Toschke, A.M. & Andler, W. Lifestyle intervention in

obese children with non-alcoholic fatty liver disease: 2-year follow-up study. Arch Dis Child 94, 437-442 (2009).

480. Pozzato, C., *et al.* Liver fat change in obese children after a 1-year nutrition-behavior intervention. *Journal of pediatric gastroenterology and nutrition* 51, 331-335 (2010).

481. Chalasani, N., *et al.* The diagnosis and management of non-alcoholic fatty liver disease: practice guideline by the American Gastroenterological Association, American Association for the Study of Liver Diseases, and American College of Gastroenterology. *Gastroenterology* 142, 1592-1609 (2012).

482. Nobili, V., *et al.* NAFLD in children: a prospective clinical-pathological study and effect of lifestyle advice. *Hepatology* 44, 458-465 (2006).

483. Nobili, V., *et al.* Metformin use in children with nonalcoholic fatty liver disease: an open-label, 24-month, observational pilot study. *Clin Ther* 30, 1168-1176 (2008).

484. Nobili, V., *et al.* Lifestyle intervention and antioxidant therapy in children with nonalcoholic fatty liver disease: a randomized, controlled trial. *Hepatology* 48, 119-128 (2008).

485. Lavine, J.E., *et al.* Effect of vitamin E or metformin for treatment of nonalcoholic fatty liver disease in children and adolescents: the TONIC randomized controlled trial. *JAMA* 305, 1659-1668 (2011).

486. Friesen, C.A. & Roberts, C.C. Cholelithiasis. Clinical characteristics in children. Case analysis and literature review. *Clin Pediatr (Phila)* 28, 294-298 (1989).

487. Holcomb, G.W., Jr., O'Neill, J.A., Jr. & Holcomb, G.W., 3rd. Cholecystitis, cholelithiasis and common duct stenosis in children and adolescents. *Annals of surgery* 191, 626-635 (1980).

488. Goodman, D.B. Cholelithiasis in persons under 25 years old. Clinicopathologic review of 96 cases. *JAMA* 236, 1731-1732 (1976).

489. Koebnick, C., *et al.* Pediatric obesity and gallstone disease. Journal of pediatric gastroenterology and nutrition 55, 328-333 (2012).

490. Mehta, S., *et al.* Clinical characteristics and risk factors for symptomatic pediatric gallbladder disease. *Pediatrics* 129, e82-88 (2012).

491. Reif, S., Sloven, D.G. & Lebenthal, E. Gallstones in children. Characterization by age, etiology, and outcome. *Am J Dis Child* 145, 105-108 (1991).

492. Kaechele, V., *et al.* Prevalence of gallbladder stone disease in obese children and adolescents: influence of the degree of obesity, sex, and pubertal development. *Journal of pediatric gastroenterology and nutrition* 42, 66-70 (2006).

493. Anand, G. & Katz, P.O. Gastroesophageal reflux disease and obesity. *Reviews in gastroenterological disorders* 8, 233-239 (2008).

494. Verhulst, S.L., *et al.* Sleep-disordered breathing in overweight and obese children and adolescents: prevalence, characteristics and the role of fat distribution. *Arch Dis Child* 92, 205-208 (2007).

495. Bonuck, K., Chervin, R.D. & Howe, L.D. Sleep-Disordered Breathing, Sleep Duration, and Childhood Overweight: A Longitudinal Cohort Study. *The Journal of Pediatrics.*

496. Krebs, N.F., *et al.* Assessment of child and adolescent overweight and obesity. *Pediatrics* 120 **Suppl** 4, S193-228 (2007).

497. Hochberg, M.C., *et al.* The association of body weight, body fatness and body fat distribution with osteoarthritis of the knee: data from the Baltimore Longitudinal Study of Aging. *J Rheumatol* 22, 488-493 (1995).

498. Hart, D.J. & Spector, T.D. The relationship of obesity, fat distribution and osteoarthritis in women in the general population: the Chingford Study. *J Rheumatol* **20**, 331-335 (1993).

499. Sandberg, M.E., *et al.* Overweight decreases the chance of achieving good response and low disease activity in early rheumatoid arthritis. *Annals of the rheumatic diseases* (2014).

500. Sandberg, M.E., *et al.* Patients with regular physical activity before onset of rheumatoid arthritis present with milder disease. *Annals of the rheumatic diseases* (2014).

501. Choi, H.K., Atkinson, K., Karlson, E.W. & Curhan, G. Obesity, weight change, hypertension, diuretic use, and risk of gout in men: the health professionals follow-up study. *Arch Intern Med* **165**, 742-748 (2005).

502. Taylor, E.D., *et al.* Orthopedic complications of overweight in children and adolescents. *Pediatrics* **117**, 2167-2174 (2006).

503. Stovitz, S.D., Pardee, P.E., Vazquez, G., Duval, S. & Schwimmer, J.B. Musculoskeletal pain in obese children and adolescents. *Acta Paediatr* **97**, 489-493 (2008).

504. Chan, G. & Chen, C.T. Musculoskeletal effects of obesity. *Current opinion in pediatrics* **21**, 65-70 (2009).

505. Pomerantz, W.J., Timm, N.L. & Gittelman, M.A. Injury patterns in obese versus nonobese children presenting to a pediatric emergency department. *Pediatrics* **125**, 681-685 (2010).

506. Kliegman, R.M., Stanton, B.M.D., St. Geme, J., Schor, N.F. & Behrman, R.E. *Nelson textbook of pediatrics*, (Saunders, 2011).

507. Dietz, W.H., Jr., Gross, W.L. & Kirkpatrick, J.A., Jr. Blount disease (tibia vara): another skeletal disorder associated with childhood obesity. *J Pediatr* **101**, 735-737 (1982).

508. Henderson, R.C. Tibia vara: a complication of adolescent obesity. *J Pediatr* **121**, 482-486 (1992).

509. Blount, W.P. Tibia vara, osteochondrosis deformans tibiae. *Current practice in orthopaedic surgery* **3**, 141-156 (1966).

510. Thompson, G.H. & Carter, J.R. Late-onset tibia vara (Blount's disease). Current concepts. *Clin Orthop Relat Res*, 24-35 (1990).

511. Davids, J.R., Huskamp, M. & Bagley, A.M. A dynamic biomechanical analysis of the etiology of adolescent tibia vara. *Journal of pediatric orthopedics* **16**, 461-468 (1996).

512. Loder, R.T., Schaffer, J.J. & Bardenstein, M.B. Late-onset tibia vara. *Journal of pediatric orthopedics* **11**, 162-167 (1991).

513. Sabharwal, S., Zhao, C. & McClemens, E. Correlation of body mass index and radiographic deformities in children with Blount disease. *J Bone Joint Surg Am* **89**, 1275-1283 (2007).

514. Henderson, R.C., Kemp, G.J. & Hayes, P.R. Prevalence of late-onset tibia vara. *Journal of pediatric orthopedics* **13**, 255-258 (1993).

515. Tachdjian, M.O. The knee and leg. in *Clinical Pediatric Orthopedics: The Art of Diagnosis and Principles of Management* (Appleton and Lange, Stamford, 1997).

516. Goulding, A., Jones, I.E., Taylor, R.W., Williams, S.M. & Manning, P.J. Bone mineral density and body composition in boys with distal forearm fractures: a dual-energy x-ray absorptiometry study. *J Pediatr* **139**, 509-515 (2001).

517. Dimitri, P., Wales, J.K. & Bishop, N. Fat and bone in children: differential effects of obesity on bone size and mass according to fracture history. *J Bone Miner Res* **25**, 527-536 (2010).

518. Wetzsteon, R.J., *et al.* Bone structure and volumetric BMD in overweight children: a longitudinal study. *J Bone Miner Res* **23**, 1946-1953 (2008).

519. Lenders, C.M., *et al.* Relation of body fat indexes to vitamin D status and deficiency among obese adolescents. *Am J Clin Nutr* **90**, 459-467 (2009).

520. Molenaar, E.A., Numans, M.E., van Ameijden, E.J. & Grobbee, D.E. [Considerable comorbidity in overweight adults: results from the Utrecht Health Project]. *Ned Tijdschr Geneeskd* **152**, 2457-2463 (2008).

521. Jemal, A., *et al.* Global cancer statistics. *CA: a cancer journal for clinicians* **61**, 69-90 (2011).

522. Brawley, O.W. Avoidable cancer deaths globally. *CA: a cancer journal for clinicians* **61**, 67-68 (2011).

523. Siegel, R., Ward, E., Brawley, O. & Jemal, A. Cancer statistics, 2011: the impact of eliminating socioeconomic and racial disparities on premature cancer deaths. *CA: a cancer journal for clinicians* **61**, 212-236 (2011).

524. Reeves, G.K., *et al.* Cancer incidence and mortality in relation to body mass index in the Million Women Study: cohort study. *BMJ* **335**, 1134 (2007).

525. Wolin, K.Y., Carson, K. & Colditz, G.A. Obesity and cancer. *The oncologist* **15**, 556-565 (2010).

526. Calle, E.E., Rodriguez, C., Walker-Thurmond, K. & Thun, M.J. Overweight, obesity, and mortality from cancer in a prospectively studied cohort of U.S. adults. *N Engl J Med* **348**, 1625-1638 (2003).

527. Bhaskaran, K., *et al.* Body-mass index and risk of 22 specific cancers: a population-based cohort study of 5.24 million UK adults. *Lancet* **384**, 755-765 (2014).

528. Wolin, K.Y., Yan, Y., Colditz, G.A. & Lee, I.M. Physical activity and colon cancer prevention: a meta-analysis. *Br J Cancer* **100**, 611-616 (2009).

529. Renehan, A.G., Tyson, M., Egger, M., Heller, R.F. & Zwahlen, M. Body-mass index and incidence of cancer: a systematic review and meta-analysis of prospective observational studies. *Lancet* **371**, 569-578 (2008).

530. Freedland, S.J. & Platz, E.A. Obesity and prostate cancer: making sense out of apparently conflicting data. *Epidemiologic reviews* **29**, 88-97 (2007).

531. Adams, T.D., *et al.* Long-term mortality after gastric bypass surgery. *N Engl J Med* **357**, 753-761 (2007).

532. Campbell, P.T., *et al.* Excess body weight and colorectal cancer risk in Canada: associations in subgroups of clinically defined familial risk of cancer. *Cancer Epidemiol Biomarkers Prev* **16**, 1735-1744 (2007).

533. Eliassen, A.H., Colditz, G.A., Rosner, B., Willett, W.C. & Hankinson, S.E. Adult weight change and risk of postmenopausal breast cancer. *JAMA* **296**, 193-201 (2006).

534. Ezzati, M., *et al.* Selected major risk factors and global and regional burden of disease. *Lancet* **360**, 1347-1360 (2002).

535. US Department of Health and Human Services. Promoting Physical Activity: A Guide for Community Action. (1999).

536. Harvard Report on Cancer Prevention. Causes of human cancer. Cancer Causes Control Vol. 1 (1998; 7 Suppl 1:S3.).

537. Kushi, L.H., *et al.* American Cancer Society Guidelines on nutrition and physical activity for cancer prevention: reducing the risk of cancer with healthy food choices and physical activity. *CA: a cancer journal for clinicians* **62**, 30-67 (2012).

538. Inoue, M., *et al.* Daily total physical activity level and total cancer risk in men and women: results from a large-scale population-based cohort study in Japan. *Am J Epidemiol* **168**, 391-403 (2008).

539. Colditz, G.A., Cannuscio, C.C. & Frazier, A.L. Physical activity and reduced risk of colon cancer: implications for prevention. *Cancer Causes Control* **8**, 649-667 (1997).

540. Dallal, C.M., *et al.* Long-term recreational physical activity and risk of invasive and in situ breast cancer: the California teachers study. *Arch Intern Med* **167**, 408-415 (2007).

541. Chao, A., *et al.* Amount, type, and timing of recreational physical activity in relation to colon and rectal cancer in older adults: the Cancer Prevention Study II Nutrition Cohort. *Cancer Epidemiol Biomarkers Prev* **13**, 2187-2195 (2004).

542. Boyle, T., Keegel, T., Bull, F., Heyworth, J. & Fritschi, L. Physical activity and risks of proximal and distal colon cancers: a systematic review and meta-analysis. *Journal of the National Cancer Institute* **104**, 1548-1561 (2012).

543. Wolin, K.Y., Yan, Y. & Colditz, G.A. Physical activity and risk of colon adenoma: a meta-analysis. *Br J Cancer* **104**, 882-885 (2011).

544. Martinez, M.E., *et al.* Leisure-time physical activity, body size, and colon cancer in women. Nurses' Health Study Research Group. *Journal of the National Cancer Institute* **89**, 948-955 (1997).

545. Rockhill, B., *et al.* A prospective study of recreational physical activity and breast cancer risk. *Arch Intern Med* **159**, 2290-2296 (1999).

546. Hu, F.B., *et al.* Adiposity as compared with physical activity in predicting mortality among women. *N Engl J Med* **351**, 2694-2703 (2004).

547. Antonelli, J.A., *et al.* Exercise and prostate cancer risk in a cohort of veterans undergoing prostate needle biopsy. *The Journal of urology* **182**, 2226-2231 (2009).

548. Patel, A.V., *et al.* Recreational physical activity and risk of prostate cancer in a large cohort of U.S. men. *Cancer Epidemiol Biomarkers Prev* **14**, 275-279 (2005).

549. McKeown-Eyssen, G. Epidemiology of colorectal cancer revisited: are serum triglycerides and/or plasma glucose associated with risk? *Cancer Epidemiol Biomarkers Prev* **3**, 687-695 (1994).

550. Giovannucci, E., *et al.* Physical activity, obesity, and risk for colon cancer and adenoma in men. *Ann Intern Med* **122**, 327-334 (1995).

551. Martinez, M.E., *et al.* Physical activity, body mass index, and prostaglandin E2 levels in rectal mucosa. *Journal of the National Cancer Institute* **91**, 950-953 (1999).

552. Maruti, S.S., Willett, W.C., Feskanich, D., Rosner, B. & Colditz, G.A. A prospective study of age-specific physical activity and premenopausal breast cancer. *Journal of the National Cancer Institute* **100**, 728-737 (2008).

553. Bernstein, L. Exercise and breast cancer prevention. *Current oncology reports* **11**, 490-496 (2009).

554. Key, T.J. Fruit and vegetables and cancer risk. *Br J Cancer* **104**, 6-11 (2011).

555. Martinez, M.E., Marshall, J.R. & Giovannucci, E. Diet and cancer prevention: the roles of observation and experimentation. *Nature reviews. Cancer* **8**, 694-703 (2008).

556. Kushi, L. & Giovannucci, E. Dietary fat and cancer. *Am J Med* **113 Suppl 9B**,

63S-70S (2002).

557. Beresford, S.A., *et al.* Low-fat dietary pattern and risk of colorectal cancer: the Women's Health Initiative Randomized Controlled Dietary Modification Trial. *JAMA* **295**, 643-654 (2006).

558. Prentice, R.L., *et al.* Low-fat dietary pattern and risk of invasive breast cancer: the Women's Health Initiative Randomized Controlled Dietary Modification Trial. *JAMA* **295**, 629-642 (2006).

559. Franceschi, S., *et al.* Dietary glycemic load and colorectal cancer risk. *Ann Oncol* **12**, 173-178 (2001).

560. Willett, W.C. Diet and cancer: one view at the start of the millennium. *Cancer Epidemiol Biomarkers Prev* **10**, 3-8 (2001).

561. Torloni, M.R., *et al.* Prepregnancy BMI and the risk of gestational diabetes: a systematic review of the literature with meta-analysis. *Obesity reviews : an official journal of the International Association for the Study of Obesity* **10**, 194-203 (2009).

562. Scott-Pillai, R., Spence, D., Cardwell, C.R., Hunter, A. & Holmes, V.A. The impact of body mass index on maternal and neonatal outcomes: a retrospective study in a UK obstetric population, 2004-2011. *BJOG : an international journal of obstetrics and gynaecology* **120**, 932-939 (2013).

563. Blomberg, M. Maternal obesity, mode of delivery, and neonatal outcome. *Obstet Gynecol* **122**, 50-55 (2013).

564. Gunatilake, R.P. & Perlow, J.H. Obesity and pregnancy: clinical management of the obese gravida. *Am J Obstet Gynecol* **204**, 106-119 (2011).

565. Abrams, B.F. & Laros, R.K., Jr. Prepregnancy weight, weight gain, and birth weight. *Am J Obstet Gynecol* **154**, 503-509 (1986).

566. Calandra, C., Abell, D.A. & Beischer, N.A. Maternal obesity in pregnancy. *Obstet Gynecol* **57**, 8-12 (1981).

567. Ehrenberg, H.M., Dierker, L., Milluzzi, C. & Mercer, B.M. Prevalence of maternal obesity in an urban center. *Am J Obstet Gynecol* **187**, 1189-1193 (2002).

568. Garbaciak, J.A., Jr., Richter, M., Miller, S. & Barton, J.J. Maternal weight and pregnancy complications. *Am J Obstet Gynecol* **152**, 238-245 (1985).

569. Gross, T., Sokol, R.J. & King, K.C. Obesity in pregnancy: risks and outcome. *Obstet Gynecol* **56**, 446-450 (1980).

570. Lu, G.C., *et al.* The effect of the increasing prevalence of maternal obesity on perinatal morbidity. *Am J Obstet Gynecol* **185**, 845-849 (2001).

571. LaCoursiere, D.Y., Bloebaum, L., Duncan, J.D. & Varner, M.W. Population-based trends and correlates of maternal overweight and obesity, Utah 1991-2001. *Am J Obstet Gynecol* **192**, 832-839 (2005).

572. Usha Kiran, T.S., Hemmadi, S., Bethel, J. & Evans, J. Outcome of pregnancy in a woman with an increased body mass index. *BJOG : an international journal of obstetrics and gynaecology* **112**, 768-772 (2005).

573. Gambineri, A., Pelusi, C., Vicennati, V., Pagotto, U. & Pasquali, R. Obesity and the polycystic ovary syndrome. *International journal of obesity and related metabolic disorders : journal of the International Association for the Study of Obesity* **26**, 883-896 (2002).

574. Panidis, D., *et al.* Obesity, weight loss, and the polycystic ovary syndrome: effect of treatment with diet and orlistat for 24 weeks on insulin resistance and androgen levels. *Fertil Steril* **89**, 899-906 (2008).

575. van der Steg, J.W., *et al.* Obesity affects spontaneous pregnancy chances in

subfertile, ovulatory women. *Hum Reprod* **23**, 324-328 (2008).
576. Gesink Law, D.C., Maclehose, R.F. & Longnecker, M.P. Obesity and time to pregnancy. *Hum Reprod* **22**, 414-420 (2007).
577. Ramlau-Hansen, C.H., *et al.* Subfecundity in overweight and obese couples. *Hum Reprod* **22**, 1634-1637 (2007).
578. Sebire, N.J., *et al.* Maternal obesity and pregnancy outcome: a study of 287,213 pregnancies in London. *International journal of obesity and related metabolic disorders : journal of the International Association for the Study of Obesity* **25**, 1175-1182 (2001).
579. Halloran, D.R., Cheng, Y.W., Wall, T.C., Macones, G.A. & Caughey, A.B. Effect of maternal weight on postterm delivery. *Journal of perinatology : official journal of the California Perinatal Association* **32**, 85-90 (2012).
580. Poobalan, A.S., Aucott, L.S., Gurung, T., Smith, W.C. & Bhattacharya, S. Obesity as an independent risk factor for elective and emergency caesarean delivery in nulliparous women--systematic review and meta-analysis of cohort studies. Obesity reviews : an official journal of the *International Association for the Study of Obesity* **10**, 28-35 (2009).
581. Gunatilake, R.P., *et al.* Predictors of failed trial of labor among women with an extremely obese body mass index. *Am J Obstet Gynecol* **209**, 562 e561-565 (2013).
582. Owens, L.A., *et al.* ATLANTIC DIP: the impact of obesity on pregnancy outcome in glucose-tolerant women. *Diabetes Care* **33**, 577-579 (2010).
583. Johnson, J.W., Longmate, J.A. & Frentzen, B. Excessive maternal weight and pregnancy outcome. *Am J Obstet Gynecol* **167**, 353-370; discussion 370-352 (1992).
584. Witter, F.R., Caulfield, L.E. & Stoltzfus, R.J. Influence of maternal anthropometric status and birth weight on the risk of cesarean delivery. *Obstet Gynecol* **85**, 947-951 (1995).
585. Perlow, J.H. & Morgan, M.A. Massive maternal obesity and perioperative cesarean morbidity. *Am J Obstet Gynecol* **170**, 560-565 (1994).
586. Hood, D.D. & Dewan, D.M. Anesthetic and obstetric outcome in morbidly obese parturients. *Anesthesiology* **79**, 1210-1218 (1993).
587. Galtier-Dereure, F., Montpeyroux, F., Boulot, P., Bringer, J. & Jaffiol, C. Weight excess before pregnancy: complications and cost. *International journal of obesity and related metabolic disorders : journal of the International Association for the Study of Obesity* **19**, 443-448 (1995).
588. Hunskaar, S. A systematic review of overweight and obesity as risk factors and targets for clinical intervention for urinary incontinence in women. *Neurourol Urodyn* **27**, 749-757 (2008).
589. Bart, S., *et al.* [Stress urinary incontinence and obesity]. *Progres en urologie : journal de l'Association francaise d'urologie et de la Societe francaise d'urologie* **18**, 493-498 (2008).
590. Subak, L.L., *et al.* Weight loss to treat urinary incontinence in overweight and obese women. *N Engl J Med* **360**, 481-490 (2009).
591. Esposito, K., *et al.* Effect of lifestyle changes on erectile dysfunction in obese men: a randomized controlled trial. *JAMA* **291**, 2978-2984 (2004).
592. Ejerblad, E., *et al.* Obesity and risk for chronic renal failure. *J Am Soc Nephrol* **17**, 1695-1702 (2006).
593. Barness, L.A., Opitz, J.M. & Gilbert-Barness, E. Obesity: genetic, molecular, and

environmental aspects. *American journal of medical genetics. Part A* **143A**, 3016-3034 (2007).

594. Mokdad, A.H., Marks, J.S., Stroup, D.F. & Gerberding, J.L. Actual causes of death in the United States, 2000. *JAMA* **291**, 1238-1245 (2004).

595. Allison, D.B., Fontaine, K.R., Manson, J.E., Stevens, J. & VanItallie, T.B. Annual deaths attributable to obesity in the United States. *JAMA* **282**, 1530-1538 (1999).

596. Mehta, N.K. & Chang, V.W. Mortality attributable to obesity among middle-aged adults in the United States. *Demography* **46**, 851-872 (2009).

597. Olshansky, S.J., *et al.* A potential decline in life expectancy in the United States in the 21st century. *N Engl J Med* **352**, 1138-1145 (2005).

598. Preston, S.H. Deadweight?--The influence of obesity on longevity. *N Engl J Med* **352**, 1135-1137 (2005).

599. Stewart, S.T., Cutler, D.M. & Rosen, A.B. Forecasting the effects of obesity and smoking on U.S. life expectancy. *N Engl J Med* **361**, 2252-2260 (2009).

600. Peeters, A., *et al.* Obesity in adulthood and its consequences for life expectancy: a life-table analysis. *Ann Intern Med* **138**, 24-32 (2003).

601. Marshall, E. Epidemiology. Public enemy number one: tobacco or obesity? *Science* **304**, 804 (2004).

602. Yan, L.L., *et al.* Midlife body mass index and hospitalization and mortality in older age. *JAMA* **295**, 190-198 (2006).

603. Gu, D., *et al.* Body weight and mortality among men and women in China. *JAMA* **295**, 776-783 (2006).

604. Adams, K.F., *et al.* Overweight, obesity, and mortality in a large prospective cohort of persons 50 to 71 years old. *N Engl J Med* **355**, 763-778 (2006).

605. Jee, S.H., *et al.* Body-mass index and mortality in Korean men and women. *N Engl J Med* **355**, 779-787 (2006).

606. McTigue, K., *et al.* Mortality and cardiac and vascular outcomes in extremely obese women. *JAMA* **296**, 79-86 (2006).

607. Freedman, D.M., Ron, E., Ballard-Barbash, R., Doody, M.M. & Linet, M.S. Body mass index and all-cause mortality in a nationwide US cohort. *International journal of obesity* **30**, 822-829 (2006).

608. Price, G.M., Uauy, R., Breeze, E., Bulpitt, C.J. & Fletcher, A.E. Weight, shape, and mortality risk in older persons: elevated waist-hip ratio, not high body mass index, is associated with a greater risk of death. *Am J Clin Nutr* **84**, 449-460 (2006).

609. Pischon, T., *et al.* General and abdominal adiposity and risk of death in Europe. *N Engl J Med* **359**, 2105-2120 (2008).

610. Prospective Studies, C., *et al.* Body-mass index and cause-specific mortality in 900 000 adults: collaborative analyses of 57 prospective studies. *Lancet* **373**, 1083-1096 (2009).

611. Flegal, K.M., Graubard, B.I., Williamson, D.F. & Gail, M.H. Cause-specific excess deaths associated with underweight, overweight, and obesity. *JAMA* **298**, 2028-2037 (2007).

612. Tobias, D.K., *et al.* Body-mass index and mortality among adults with incident type 2 diabetes. *N Engl J Med* **370**, 233-244 (2014).

613. Kramer, C.K., Zinman, B. & Retnakaran, R. Are metabolically healthy overweight and obesity benign conditions?: A systematic review and meta-analysis. *Ann Intern Med* **159**, 758-769 (2013).

614. Flegal, K.M., Kit, B.K., Orpana, H. & Graubard, B.I. Association of all-cause

mortality with overweight and obesity using standard body mass index categories: a systematic review and meta-analysis. *JAMA* **309**, 71-82 (2013).

615. Mokdad, A.H., Marks, J.S., Stroup, D.F. & Gerberding, J.L. Correction: actual causes of death in the United States, 2000. *JAMA* **293**, 293-294 (2005).

616. Flegal, K.M., Graubard, B.I., Williamson, D.F. & Gail, M.H. Excess deaths associated with underweight, overweight, and obesity. *JAMA* **293**, 1861-1867 (2005).

617. Boggs, D.A., *et al.* General and abdominal obesity and risk of death among black women. *N Engl J Med* **365**, 901-908 (2011).

618. Berrington de Gonzalez, A., *et al.* Body-mass index and mortality among 1.46 million white adults. *N Engl J Med* **363**, 2211-2219 (2010).

619. Zheng, W., *et al.* Association between body-mass index and risk of death in more than 1 million Asians. *N Engl J Med* **364**, 719-729 (2011).

620. Mark, D.H. Deaths attributable to obesity. *JAMA* **293**, 1918-1919 (2005).

621. Tsai, A.G. & Wadden, T.A. In the clinic: obesity. *Ann Intern Med* **159**, ITC3-1-ITC3-15; quiz ITC13-16 (2013).

622. Wildman, R.P., *et al.* The obese without cardiometabolic risk factor clustering and the normal weight with cardiometabolic risk factor clustering: prevalence and correlates of 2 phenotypes among the US population (NHANES 1999-2004). *Arch Intern Med* **168**, 1617-1624 (2008).

623. Bell, J.A., *et al.* The Natural Course of Healthy Obesity Over 20 Years. *Journal of the American College of Cardiology* **65**, 101-102 (2015).

624. Chen, Y., *et al.* Association between body mass index and cardiovascular disease mortality in east Asians and south Asians: pooled analysis of prospective data from the Asia Cohort Consortium. *BMJ* **347**, f5446 (2013).

625. Gregg, E.W., *et al.* Secular trends in cardiovascular disease risk factors according to body mass index in US adults. *JAMA* **293**, 1868-1874 (2005).

626. Alley, D.E. & Chang, V.W. The changing relationship of obesity and disability, 1988-2004. *JAMA* **298**, 2020-2027 (2007).

627. Calle, E.E., Teras, L.R. & Thun, M.J. Obesity and mortality. *N Engl J Med* **353**, 2197-2199 (2005).

628. Barry, V.W., *et al.* Fitness vs. fatness on all-cause mortality: a meta-analysis. *Progress in cardiovascular diseases* **56**, 382-390 (2014).

629. Stevens, J., Cai, J., Evenson, K.R. & Thomas, R. Fitness and fatness as predictors of mortality from all causes and from cardiovascular disease in men and women in the lipid research clinics study. *Am J Epidemiol* **156**, 832-841 (2002).

630. Grover, S.A., *et al.* Years of life lost and healthy life-years lost from diabetes and cardiovascular disease in overweight and obese people: a modelling study. *The lancet. Diabetes & endocrinology* (2014).

631. Fontaine, K.R., Redden, D.T., Wang, C., Westfall, A.O. & Allison, D.B. Years of life lost due to obesity. *JAMA* **289**, 187-193 (2003).

632. Finkelstein, E.A., Trogdon, J.G., Cohen, J.W. & Dietz, W. Annual medical spending attributable to obesity: payer-and service-specific estimates. *Health Aff (Millwood)* **28**, w822-831 (2009).

633. Trasande, L. & Chatterjee, S. The impact of obesity on health service utilization and costs in childhood. *Obesity* **17**, 1749-1754 (2009).

634. Trasande, L., Liu, Y., Fryer, G. & Weitzman, M. Effects of childhood obesity on hospital care and costs, 1999-2005. *Health Aff (Millwood)* **28**, w751-760 (2009).

635. Cawley, J. & Meyerhoefer, C. The medical care costs of obesity: an instrumental variables approach. *Journal of health economics* **31**, 219-230 (2012).

636. Quesenberry, C.P., Jr., Caan, B. & Jacobson, A. Obesity, health services use, and health care costs among members of a health maintenance organization. *Arch Intern Med* **158**, 466-472 (1998).

637. Thompson, D., Brown, J.B., Nichols, G.A., Elmer, P.J. & Oster, G. Body mass index and future healthcare costs: a retrospective cohort study. *Obes Res* **9**, 210-218 (2001).

Printed in Great Britain
by Amazon